The Temporal Bone

John I. Lane
Robert J. Witte

The Temporal Bone

An Imaging Atlas

Springer

John I. Lane, MD
Consultant, Department of Radiology,
Mayo Clinic
Associate Professor of Radiology,
College of Medicine, Mayo Clinic
200 First Street SW.,
Rochester MN 55905
USA
Lane.john@mayo.edu

Robert J. Witte, MD
Consultant, Department of Radiology,
Mayo Clinic
Associate Professor of Radiology,
College of Medicine, Mayo Clinic
200 First Street SW.,
Rochester MN 55905
USA
Witte.robert@mayo.edu

ISBN: 978-3-662-50108-5 ISBN: 978-3-642-02210-4 (eBook)

DOI: 10.1007/978-3-642-02210-4

Springer Heidelberg Dordrecht London New York

Cover design: eStudio Calamar, Figueres/Berlin

Printed on acid-free paper

Springer is part of Springer Science+Business Media (www.springer.com)

Additional material to this book can be downloaded from http://extras.springer.com

Preface

The study of the temporal bone represents one of the most formidable challenges in clinical anatomy secondary to the small size of its component structures and the difficulties entailed in gaining adequate exposure while minimizing the destructive process of anatomical dissection. In this atlas we employ the use of CT and MR microscopy scanners, commonly used in research laboratories to image small animals such as mice or rats, to study the temporal bones harvested from human cadavers. Although these imaging techniques currently cannot compete with high power light microscopy (let alone even higher power microscopic tools) and can only achieve resolutions of 20–80 μm, they allow us to obtain an isotropic volumetric acquisition that can be reconstructed in any plane of section with no additional tissue destruction. The volumetric nature of the acquisitions also allows the reconstruction of 3D images that are ideal for demonstrating the complex anatomical relationships of the middle and inner ear. These relationships are often most effectively portrayed in temporal bone anatomy publications by the use of medical art work. In the anatomy section of this book (Chap. 2), we have attempted to replace the standard medical illustrations of the middle and inner ear with 3D reconstructions generated from imaging microscopy data. We believe that the use of 3D image postprocessing, another advantage of volumetric acquisitions, facilitates understanding of the unique anatomical relationships of the miniscule structures that compose the temporal bone. Several temporal bone labs have done similar work with digitization of microtomed histological section, but these techniques are limited by microtome artifacts and the complexities of digitizing histological sections.

The microimaging techniques we have employed produce images that are similar in appearance to those acquired in clinical medicine using state-of-the-art multidetector computed tomography and high field magnetic resonance imaging. In the Multiplanar Atlas section of this book (Chap. 3) we have endeavored to carefully compare images of preserved cadaver temporal bone specimens acquired with CT microscopy at 20 μm and 9.4 T MR microscopy at 78 μm with those acquired with clinical imaging equipment used in our everyday radiology practice. Additionally, image review using multiplanar reconstructions and maximum intensity projections are useful in demonstrating complex anatomical relationships of the middle and inner ear to better effect. In the Advanced Imaging Applications section of this book (Chap. 4) we have focused on the utility of these postprocessing techniques. We have also provided a Temporal Bone Anatomy Tool on CD that will permit the user to scroll through the CT and MR microscopy datasets in three orthogonal planes on a desktop personal computer. Chapter 5 contains a brief introduction on how to use the Anatomy Tool.

It is our hope that applying these microscopic imaging techniques to the study of the temporal bone will assist us in achieving greater degrees of diagnostic accuracy using our current clinical imaging tools. In addition, we believe that familiarity with the imaging appearance of the temporal bone at this level of anatomical detail will provide the clinical imager with the incentive to push for greater degrees of resolution from our current and future clinical imaging equipment. Ultimately, improved image resolution and more accurate image interpretation will lead to better care of our patients.

Rochester, Minnesota, USA

John I. Lane, MD
Robert J. Witte, MD

Acknowledgments

This book would not have been possible without the assistance so many colleagues; we fear to mention any of them for risk of omitting even one. A special thanks is owed to Bill and Miriam Hanson at the University of North Carolina, Chapel Hill for making available their work on MR microscopy of the temporal bone that was such a critical piece of this atlas and for their gracious North Carolina hospitality. Thanks to Eric Ritman, PhD and his laboratory personnel for their assistance with acquiring all of the microCT work included in this book. Years of effort went into the postprocessing of these imaging volumes as well as the development of the Temporal Bone Anatomy Tutorial CD included with this book. Much of this was done at the Biomedical Imaging Resource (BIR) under the direction of Richard Robb, PhD. This work was overseen by Jon Camp with the able assistance of Phil Edwards. The CD animation and user interface was developed by Mark Korinek and Ron Karwoski.

Our media support department played a critical role in the subsequent postprocessing phase, enhancing the images produced in the BIR. Special thanks goes to Tristan Cummings and Paul Honermann for all their hard work down the home stretch.

We wish to acknowlege the contributions of our colleagues at Siemens Medical Solutions, in particular Kevin Johnson, RT and Brad Bolster, PhD for their assistance in acquiring the 3T MR images used in this book. We thank Cynthia McCollough, PhD and her associates at the Clinical Investigation Center at the Mayo Clinic Rochester for their support utilizing the MDCT for temporal bone work.

Colin Driscoll, MD of the Neurotology section of the Department of Otolaryngology at the Mayo Clinic Rochester was instrumental in initiating the use of imaging microscopy in the study of the temporal bone at our institution. We appreciate his invitation to participate in this work so many years ago. He and his colleagues, Brian Neff, MD and Charles Beatty, MD, have been a pleasure to work with in both the clinical and the research realms. We appreciate all the encouragment we have received for completing this project from our audiology colleagues, including Robert Brey, Jon Shallop, and Christopher Bauch. Last, but by no means least, we thank our spouses (Mary Frances Lane and Deborah Witte) and children (Erin, Brigid, John and Moira Lane; Matthew and Nathan Witte) for all their patience and understanding during the production of this book.

This work is dedicated to patients with hearing and vestibular impairment, particularly all those who have presented over the years to the Mayo Clinic Rochester. It is our hope that this work will contribute to the education and training of scientists and health care professionals who seek to further our understanding and treatment of these particular maladies. We have been endowed with many gifts, not least among them our abilities to hear and maintain balance. Our appreciation of the world around us is dependent on these sensations. The loss of these faculties can be particularly debilitating. We appreciate the opportunity to assist our clinical colleagues in the evaluation of these patients and to contribute, in our own small way, toward any possible restoration or improvement in their condition. The science and art of medicine has now progressed to the point where many of the 4,000 children born deaf each year in the USA can have their hearing restored through cochlear implantation. Such a child, born into a world of utter silence, never to hear her mother call her name or sing her a lullaby, can now be made to hear. We consider it a great privilege to play a part in these modern day miracles. *Deo Gratias*.

Rochester, Minnesota, USA

John I. Lane, MD
Robert J. Witte, MD

Contents

1 **Imaging Technique** 1
Imaging Microscopy 1
CT Microscopy 1
MR Microscopy 1
Clinical Imaging 2
Multidetector CT 2
High Field MR 2
Postprocessing 3
References 5

2 **Anatomy** 7
Surface Anatomy 7
Skin Surface 7
Bone Surface 7
Bony External Auditory Canal and Tympanic Membrane 9
Middle Ear Space 9
The Auditory Ossicles 11
The Inner Ear 11
Reference 28

3 **Multiplanar Atlas** 29
Temporal Bone Imaging: Historical Perspectives 29
The Axial Plane (in the Plane of the Lateral Semicircular Canal) 30
The Coronal Plane (Perpendicular to the Plane of the Lateral Semicircular Canal) 40
Pöschl Plane (Short Axis Plane of the Temporal Bone) 51
Stenvers Plane (Long Axis Plane of the Temporal Bone) 64
References 74

4 **Advanced Imaging Applications** 75
References 96

5 Imaging Microscopy of the Temporal Bone: An Anatomy Tutorial . . . 97
Introduction . . . 97
Temporal Bone Anatomy Tool . . . 97
Virtual Endoscopy Video Player . . . 97

Glossary . . . 99

Index . . . 107

1 Imaging Technique

Imaging Microscopy

The gold standard for studying temporal bone anatomy has been histological sectioning by microtome following chemical fixation and deossification of the temporal bone specimen. This process introduces significant artifacts visible even at low power magnification. Although imaging microscopy cannot compete with histology at higher powers of magnification (i.e., the cellular level), resolution at the 20–100 μm level is achievable, allowing study of the temporal bone without the aforementioned artifacts induced by fixation and sectioning.

CT Microscopy

Computed tomography (CT) microscopy has been primarily used in the imaging of small animals in the research laboratory. There are several obvious advantages to imaging microscopy in the study of the temporal bone compared with standard microtomed histological preparations. MicroCT avoids significant tissue destruction and artifacts introduced during the sectioning process such as fractures, soft tissue tears, fluid, blood or bone dust in the pneumatized spaces, variable section thickness, and wrinkling, which can occur during the mounting process. Specimen preparation was critical to acquiring the best possible imaging dataset. Despite a careful technique, we encountered small amounts of fluid and bone dust in the middle ear space. Air–bone interfaces also caused some minor beam-hardening artifact.

The temporal bone specimen used in this atlas was harvested from a male cadaver using the block technique, as described by Gulya [1]. The specimen had to be further reduced in size to a maximal diameter of 2.5 cm and to 4 cm in length in order to fit properly in the microCT scanner. The specimen was scanned without decalcification or additional fixation. The microCT scanning technique used to produce the images in this atlas has been previously described in the literature [2]. MicroCT scanning differs from clinical scanning in that the object is rotated between the tube and camera, which are stationary. The specimen is placed on a rotating stage, which turns 360° about its vertical axis in 0.5° increments. At each angle an X-ray exposure is recorded on the charge-coupled device (CCD) camera. A single acquisition using a 20-μm slice thickness will cover approximately 2 cm of tissue. Our specimen was scanned in two acquisitions, each taking 8 h at 35 KV and 50 mAs. The two volume acquisitions were then combined using the Analyze 3-D voxel registration program, as described by Hanson et al. and Camp et al. [3, 4]. The first image volume was padded with zero-valued voxels to enlarge the volume enough to contain the entire reassembled volume. The region of overlap between the two acquisitions was used to automatically register the second acquisition to the first. Then, an appropriate "crossover" section was determined, and the whole volume assembled. The entire volume dataset consisted of 20 μm cubic voxels.

MR Microscopy

Magnetic resonance microscopy, like CT microscopy, has been primarily used in the imaging of small animals and pathological specimens in the research laboratory. It also provides many of the same advantages as microCT in the study of the temporal bone compared with standard microtomed histological preparations.

J. I. Lane, R. J. Witte, *The Temporal Bone,* DOI: 10.1007/978-3-642-02210-4_1,

However, because air and cortical bone are virtually devoid of water protons, they generate no significant signal on MR imaging. Clinically, this prevents any meaningful imaging of the naturally aerated portions of the temporal bone. These air spaces must be filled with fluid in order for the contents of the middle ear to be studied with microMR. Specimen preparation for microMR is even more critical than for microCT in acquiring the best possible imaging dataset. Any air within the specimen can significantly degrade image quality secondary to susceptibility artifact. It is important to displace all of the air within and surrounding the specimen with fluid before scanning. This renders all aerated portions of the specimen visible on the T2-weighted acquisition.

The naturally-occurring fluid (endolymph and perilymph) that surrounds and fills the membranous structures of the inner ear within the bony labyrinth provide the T2 signal necessary to resolve the lower signal membranes on MR microscopy, most of which are currently not visible using clinical in vivo imaging.

The adult human specimen used in this atlas was obtained from the National Temporal Bone Bank, Massachusetts Eye and Ear Infirmary (courtesy of Dr. Saumil Merchant). The specimen preparation and scanning technique have been previously published [5]. The specimen was fixed 8 h postmortem in 4% phosphate buffered formalin 2 years before scanning. In preparation for scanning, it was placed in 0.1 M phosphate buffer (pH 7.4) for 2 months to remove the formalin that can degrade MR images. The bone was trimmed to reduce the size as much as possible and hence decrease the field of view (FOV), which is directly related to final voxel size. The final size allowed the field to be 40 × 40 × 40 mm in the 512 × 512 × 512 data set (40,000 μm/512 = 78.1 μm isotropic voxels). Five days before data acquisition, the bone was placed in a dilute gadolinium solution (1:500 with 0.1 M phosphate buffer) and this solution was changed daily. The middle ear cavity was opened at the tegmen to allow any trapped air to be replaced with the contrast solution. Before data acquisition, the specimen, along with fresh contrast solution, was placed in the barrel of a 25-cc syringe modified with plungers at both ends. Care was taken to express all visible air bubbles out through a 25-gauge needle inserted through the wall of the syringe. The specimen was scanned using a 3D fast spin-echo technique for a period of 13 h on a 9.4 T magnet at the Center for In Vivo Microscopy, Duke University (acquisition parameters: TR/TE, 100 ms/6.5 ms; FOV, 40 × 40 × 40 mm; matrix, 512 × 512 × 512; bandwidth, 62.5 kHz). The entire volume dataset consisted of 78-μm cubic voxels.

Clinical Imaging

Multidetector CT

Since the advent of CT, the physical limitations of gantry angle and patient positioning have largely restricted the plane of imaging in temporal bone to the standard axial and coronal orientations. However, most anatomical structures of the middle and inner ear are not optimally depicted in these planes. In the days of temporal bone polytomography, oblique projections in the short and long axis of the temporal bone (Pöschl and Stenvers planes respectively) were often obtained to better visualize some of these structures. Recent advances in multidetector CT (MDCT) technology have allowed the acquisition of volumetric data with isotropic voxels that permit image reconstruction in any plane of section [6].

Multidetector CT images of the temporal bone included in this book were all performed on a 64-slice scanner (Siemens Medical Solutions, Erlangen, Germany) in the direct axial plane using helical technique (120 kV, 350 mA, pitch of 0.85, rotation time 1 s, slice thickness 0.4 mm, matrix 512 × 512). The scanner consists of 32 rows of detectors and utilizes a "wobbling focal spot," effectively producing 64 detectors. The subject's head was placed in a neutral position without chin tilt. The dataset was reconstructed in a 70 mm FOV yielding a voxel size of 0.4 × 0.4 × 0.4 mm.

High Field MR

Because of the lack of sufficient numbers of hydrogen protons in air and bone, MR imaging of the temporal bone is limited to the fluid-containing structures of the inner ear, unless significant amounts of pathological fluid or soft tissue occupies the normally aerated middle ear. Visualization of the fluid-filled structures of the inner ear has been limited to the detection of normal fluid signal intensity within the bony labyrinth on 1.5 or 3T MR imaging. 3D T2-weighted acquisitions provide the highest image resolution currently available. These

3D sequences, to include constructive interference in the steady state (CISS) or fast spin-echo (FSE) techniques, provide excellent depiction of the nerves within the internal auditory canal as well as the fluid within the labyrinth, but attempts to image the ducts and sacs of the membranous labyrinth have been compromised by susceptibility banding artifact in the case of gradient-echo acquisitions and image blurring inherent to FSE sequences [7].

We have achieved limited success in visualizing some elements of the membranous labyrinth using a recently developed modification of the T2 FSE technique [8]. With this 3D variable flip-angle FSE (3D VFA FSE) technique, the flip angle of the refocusing pulses is not fixed at a constant value (e.g., 180°), but is instead modulated according to a predetermined schedule, which is calculated on the basis of the desired image contrast properties [9–13]. The use of the VFA evolution has several important benefits for temporal bone imaging. As designed, this technique has the effect of reducing the change in signal intensity through the echo train, allowing longer echo trains and thus enabling a high-resolution single slab isotropic acquisition in a clinically feasible scanning time. This more consistent echo-to-echo signal intensity has the additional benefit of reducing blurring, especially in tissues with relatively short T2. Furthermore, because smaller flip angles are used, the radiofrequency heating, as measured by the specific absorption rate (SAR), is substantially reduced, enabling applications at 3T without the acquisition time penalty normally associated with standard FSE technique at that field strength.

For the 3D VFA FSE acquisitions used in this book, a pseudo-steady-state flip angle evolution at 130° was chosen to obtain the high signal-to-noise ratio required for higher spatial resolution. By using this schedule, the flip angle quickly transitions to and maintains a flip angle of 130° for each echo train. This allowed relatively long echo trains (37 for these acquisitions) while staying within clinically allowed SAR limits.

The 3T MR images presented in this book were all acquired on a 3T MR imaging system (Magnetom Trio [TIM System]; Siemens Medical Solutions, Erlangen, Germany) with a 7-cm loop coil placed over the left external auditory canal of a single healthy volunteer. The 3D VFA FSE technique was used in the standard axial and coronal planes in addition to two oblique planes acquired along the short axis (Pöschl plane) and long axis (Stenvers plane) of the temporal bone. Images were acquired with a 6-cm FOV, 202 × 256 matrix, and 0.32-mm partitions, yielding nearly 0.3-mm isotropic spatial resolution. Images were further interpolated in-plane to approximately 0.14 × 0.12 mm. TR and effective TE were 1,400 ms and 131 ms respectively, yielding an acquisition time of approximately 11.5 min.

Postprocessing

All volumetric acquisitions were reconstructed in the axial (plane of the lateral semicircular canal), coronal (perpendicular to the lateral semicircular canal), Pöschl (short axis of the petrous segment), and Stenvers (long axis of the petrous segment) planes from a single volumetric acquisition with the exception of the 3T MR acquisitions. These sections were obtained in four planes of acquisition to achieve the highest degree of in-plane resolution available and thus avoid any reconstruction artifacts.

MicroCT images selected for the Multiplanar Atlas (Chap. 3) and Advanced Imaging Applications (Chap. 4) sections of the book were carefully reviewed for the presence of bone dust or retained fluid within or around the periphery of the temporal bone specimen. These areas of preparation artifact were photographically masked to match the attenuation of adjacent air-containing portions of the temporal bone. No other photographic alterations were made to these microscopy source images.

Additional multiplanar reconstructions (MPRs) and maximum intensity projections (MIPs) were reconstructed on a standard workstation (Siemens Wizard). 3D MIP images from the 3T MR scanner were reconstructed on the same workstation. 3D images from the MDCT scanner were reconstructed on a Terra Recon workstation (Houston, TX, USA). Some of the 3D images from the MDCT dataset were reconstructed after color segmentation of the bony labyrinth to provide additional detail of the inner ear structures in relation to the surface anatomy of the left temporal bone. These images have been used to indicate the approximate planes of reconstruction that precede each plane of section in the Multiplanar Atlas (Chap. 3).

3D reconstructions from the microimaging datasets used in the Anatomy section (Chap. 2) of the book were all generated using the Analyze volume-rendering module. The original microCT or microMR images were reviewed and then each anatomical structure or space was color-segmented to provide easily recognizable distinctions between structures

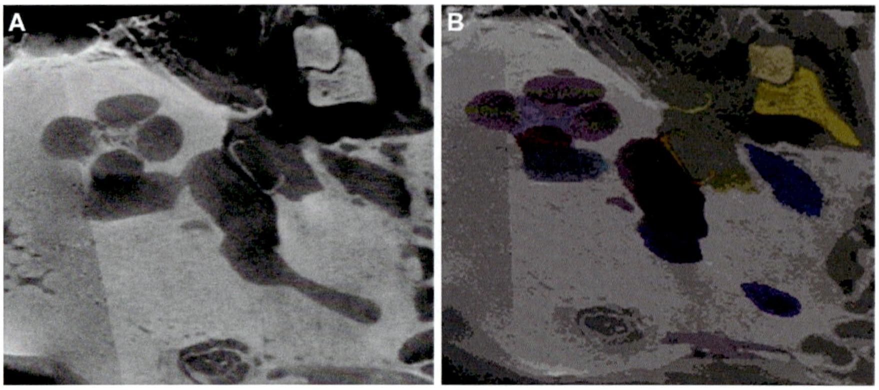

Fig. 1 CT microscopy. (**a**) Twenty-micrometer axial microCT section of the cadaver temporal bone at the level of the oval window. (**b**) Similar section with color segmentation of the anatomical structures

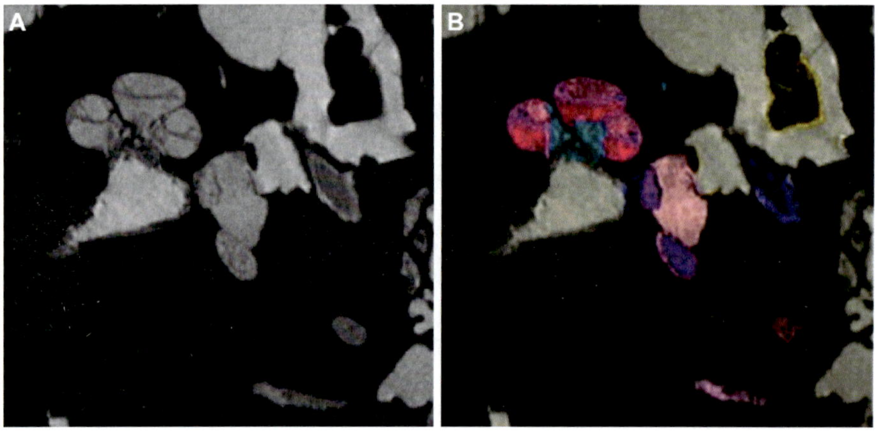

Fig. 2 MR microscopy. (**a**) Seventy-eight-micrometer axial 9.4 T microMR section of the cadaver temporal bone at the level of the oval window. (**b**) Similar section with color segmentation of the anatomical structures

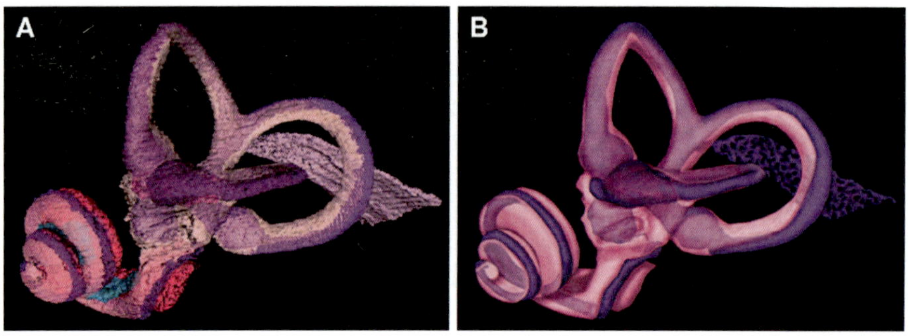

Fig. 3 Membranous labyrinth. (**a**) 3D reconstruction of the membranous labyrinth in the lateral projection from the color-segmented microMR dataset. (**b**) Medical illustrator's enhancement of the original reconstruction

(Figs. 1, 2). 3D reconstructions were then generated from the segmented data. These images were enhanced using standard photographic software, being careful not to alter the anatomical accuracy of the original image (Figs. 3, 4). In a limited number of instances, the medical artists added details to the 3D images generated for the Anatomy chapter that were not included in the original reconstructions. For example, the harvesting of the cadaver temporal bone used for microMR required sectioning the nerves in the internal auditory canal. When demonstrating the anatomy of the internal auditory canal, the artists recreated the intracanalicular segments of these nerves to show them in continuity with their respective intratemporal segments.

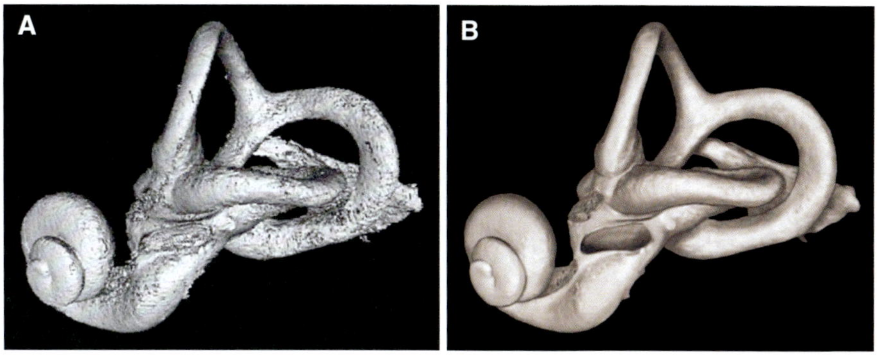

Fig. 4 Bony labyrinth. (**a**) 3D reconstruction of the bony labyrinth in the lateral projection from the microCT dataset. (**b**) Medical illustrator's enhancement of the original reconstruction

References

1. Gulya AJ Anatomy of the Temporal Bone With Surgical Implications. Informa Healthcare USA, New York, NY, 2007, 356 pp
2. Lane J, Witte R, Driscoll C, Camp J, Robb R. Imaging microscopy of the middle and inner ear: Part I: CT microscopy. *Clin Anat* 2004;17:607–612
3. Hanson D, Robb R, Aharon S, Augustine K, Cameron B. New software toolkits for comprehensive visualization and analysis of three-dimensional multimodal biomedical images. *J Digit Imaging* 1997;10:1–2
4. Camp J, Robb R. A novel binning method for improved accuracy and speed of volume image coregistration using normalized mutual information. *Proc SPIE* 1999;3661:24–31
5. Lane JI, Witte RJ, Henson OW, Driscoll CL, Camp J, Robb RA. Imaging microscopy of the middle and inner ear: Part II: MR microscopy. *Clin Anat* 2005;18:409–415
6. Lane J, Lindell E, Witte R, DeLone D, Driscoll C. Middle and inner ear: improved depiction with multiplanar reconstruction of volumetric CT data. *Radiographics* 2006;26:115–124
7. Lane J, Ward H, Witte R, Bernstein M, Driscoll C. 3T imaging of the cochlear nerve and labyrinth in cochlear-implant candidates: 3D fast recovery fast spin-echo versus 3D constructive interference in the steady state techniques. *AJNR Am J Neuroradiol* 2004;25:618–622
8. Lane J, Witte R, Bolster B, Bernstein M, Johnson K, Morris J. State of the art: 3T imaging of the membranous labyrinth. *AJNR Am J Neuroradiol* 2008;29:1436–1440
9. Mugler J, III, Kiefer B, Brookeman J. Three-dimensional T2-weighted imaging of the brain using very long spin-echo trains. *Proceedings of the 8th Annual Scientific Meeting of the International Society for Magnetic Resonance in Medicine*. Denver, CO; 2000;pp 687
10. Le Roux P, Hinks RS. Stabilization of echo amplitudes in FSE sequences. *Magn Reson Med* 1993;30:183–190
11. Alsop DC. The sensitivity of low flip angle RARE imaging. *Magn Reson Med* 1997;37:176–184
12. Hennig J, Weigel M, Scheffler K. Multiecho sequences with variable refocusing flip angles: optimization of signal behavior using smooth transitions between pseudo steady states (TRAPS). *Magn Reson Med* 2003;49: 527–535
13. Busse RF, Hariharan H, Vu A, Brittain JH. Fast spin echo sequences with very long echo trains: design of variable refocusing flip angle schedules and generation of clinical T2 contrast. *Magn Reson Med* 2006;55:1030–1037

2 Anatomy

As stated in Chap. 1, we attempt to graphically portray the 3D anatomy of the temporal bone directly from volumetric imaging data acquired from research and clinical MR and CT scanners. It is our intent to offer a temporal bone anatomy atlas that accurately demonstrates clinically important anatomical details without primarily relying on the medical artist. It is not our intent to present an exhaustive written description of temporal bone anatomy. There are timeless anatomical texts (e.g., Gray's Anatomy) with which we have no desire to compete. Where we believe we can make a contribution to anatomical and medical education is in the graphic presentation of this anatomy in a form that is as true to the object of our study as is currently possible. For the sake of uniformity, all images will focus on the left temporal bone.

At the end of this book, we have included a Glossary. All structures that appear in italics in the brief anatomical description of the temporal bone that follows below also appear in the Glossary. Any abbreviations used in the Multiplanar Atlas chapter are also listed along side the definition of the structure in the Glossary.

Surface Anatomy

Skin Surface

The external ear or *pinna* is composed of a skin-covered cartilaginous appendage consisting of the helix, antihelix, tragus, antitragus, and a noncartilaginous lobule or ear lobe (Fig. 1). The depression between ridges of the helix and antihelix is the navicular fossa. The cartilaginous portion of the external auditory canal (EAC) opens deep and posterior to the tragus.

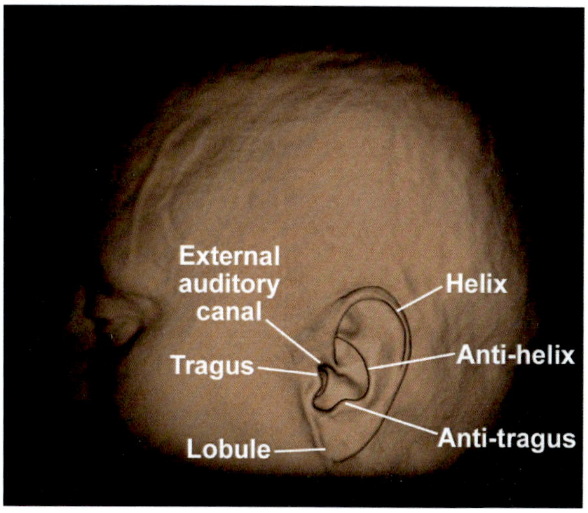

Fig. 1 External ear. 3D skin surface reconstruction of the multidetector CT (MDCT) dataset. Note anatomical landmarks of the external ear (pinna) and external auditory canal

Bone Surface

The temporal bone consists of five parts: the squamous, tympanic, mastoid, petrous, and styloid portions. The lateral surface of the temporal bone is composed of the thin squamous portion, the tympanic portion (curved plate of bone lying below the squama and in front of the mastoid process), and the mastoid portion, forming the posterior part of the lateral surface and containing an inferior conical projection (mastoid process) (Fig. 2).

The posteromedial surface is composed of the petrous portion of the temporal bone, a pyramidal shaped process wedged in at the base of the skull between the sphenoid and occipital bones and containing the orifices of the *internal auditory canal* (IAC), *cochlear aqueduct*, and *vestibular aqueduct* (Fig. 3).

J. I. Lane, R. J. Witte, *The Temporal Bone*, DOI: 10.1007/978-3-642-02210-4_2,

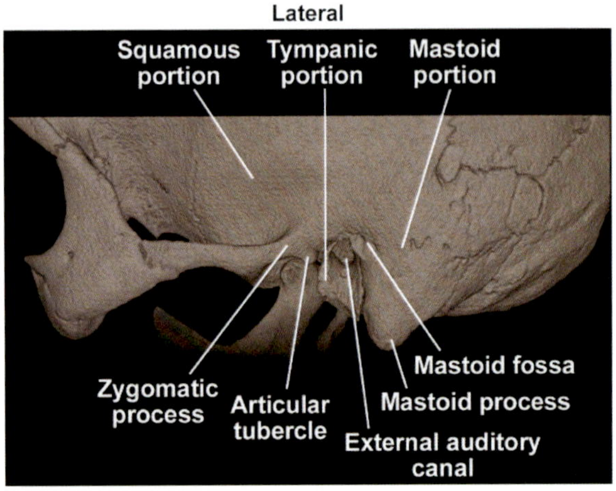

Fig. 2 Temporal bone lateral surface. 3D bone surface reconstruction of the MDCT dataset. Note *three* portions (squamous, tympanic, and mastoid) of the temporal bone comprising its lateral surface

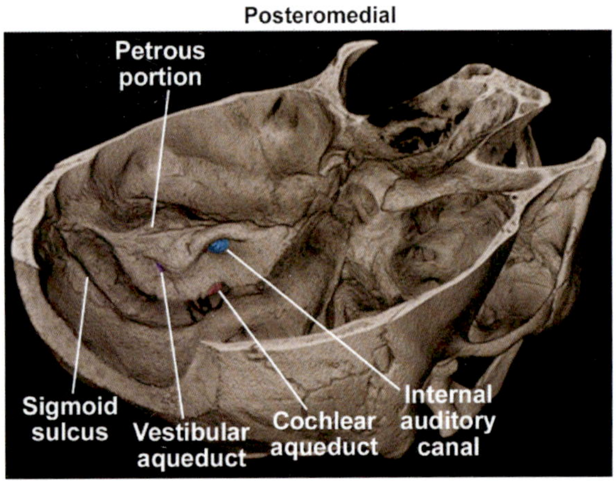

Fig. 3 Temporal bone posteromedial surface. 3D bone surface reconstruction of the MDCT dataset. Note the anatomical relationship among the openings of the internal auditory canal (*blue*), the cochlear aqueduct (*pink*), and the vestibular aqueduct (*purple*)

The petrous portion also forms the superior surface of the temporal bone as well (Fig. 4). Near the center is the *arcuate eminence*, an anatomical and surgical landmark that identifies the location of the superior semicircular canal. Anterior and lateral to the eminence, is the thin layer of bone separating the middle ear space from the middle cranial fossa, the *tegmen tympani*.

The inferior surface of the temporal bone is composed of the undersurfaces of the petrous, mastoid, tympanic, and styloid portions. Surface landmarks include the styloid process, *stylomastoid foramen of the facial nerve*, openings of the *carotid canal* and *jugular foramen*, and the tip of the mastoid process (Fig. 5).

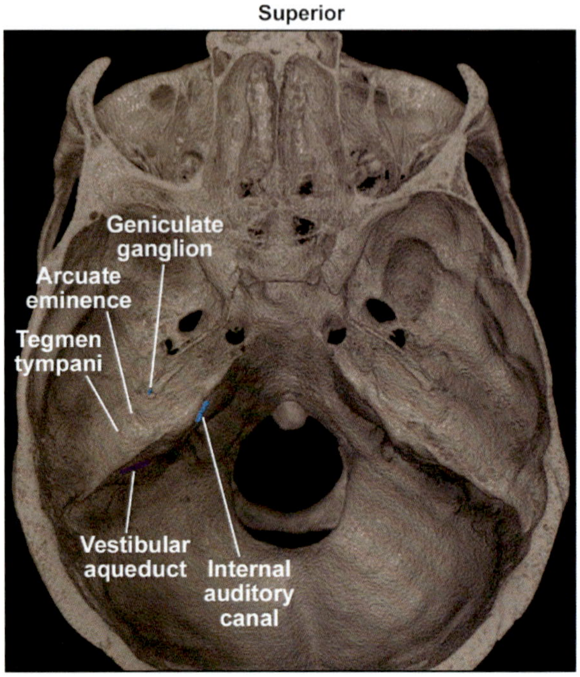

Fig. 4 Temporal bone superior surface. 3D bone surface reconstruction of the MDCT dataset. Note the relationship between the internal auditory canal (*blue*) and opening of the vestibular aqueduct (*purple*). Arcuate eminence marks the location of the superior semicircular canal. Bony covering of the geniculate ganglion of the 7th nerve is dehiscent, a normal variant

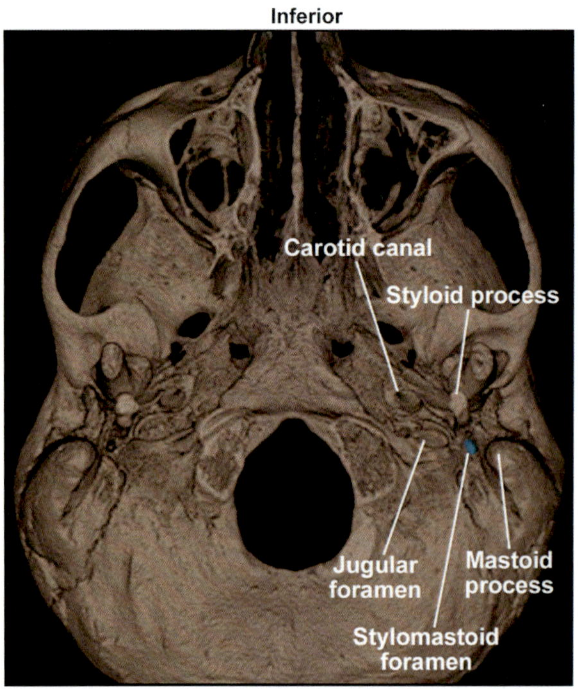

Fig. 5 Temporal bone inferior surface. 3D bone surface reconstruction of the MDCT dataset. Note the anatomical landmarks of the inferior surface of the petrous portion of the temporal bone. Note the relationship between the stylomastoid foramen of the facial nerve (*blue*) and the base of the styloid process

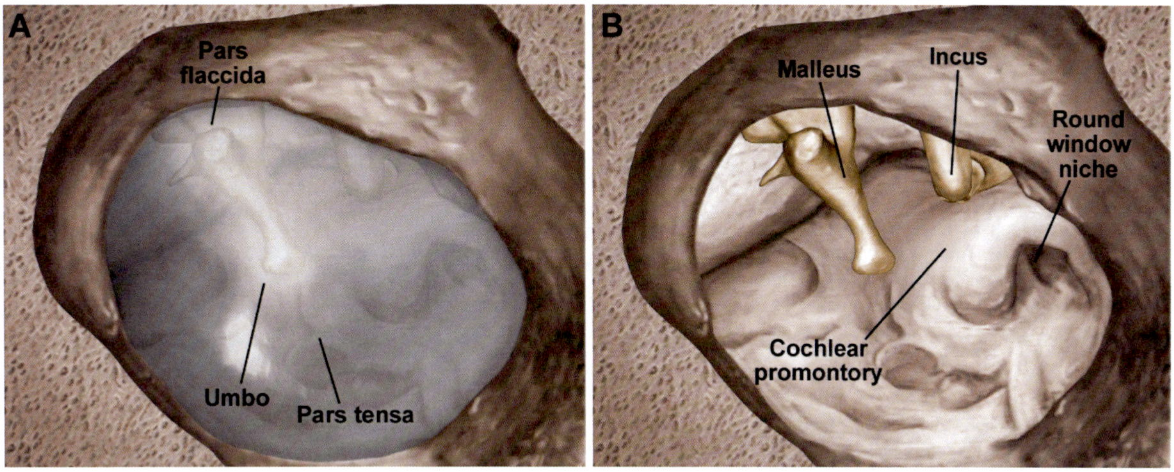

Fig. 6 Otoscopic perspective through the external auditory canal. 3D reconstruction of the microMR dataset. (**a**) View of the middle ear through the intact tympanic membrane (TM), which is lax superiorly (pars flaccida) because of a defect in the bony ring to which it is attached, and more taut inferiorly (pars tensa). Note the central depression at the manubrial attachment (umbo). (**b**) View of the middle ear with the TM removed demonstrates lower segments of the malleus and incus. Note the relationship between the cochlear promontory and the round window niche

Bony External Auditory Canal and Tympanic Membrane

The *tympanic membrane* (TM) transmits sound waves traveling through the EAC to the middle ear ossicles by way of mechanical vibration. Its outer circumference forms a fibrocartilaginous ring that is fixed at the inner edge of the EAC in the tympanic sulcus. This sulcus is deficient superiorly (*notch of Rivinus*). The triangular segment of the TM adjacent to the notch is lax and thin (*pars flaccida*); the remainder is thick and taut (*pars tensa*). Its attachment to the *manubrium* of the *malleus* draws the TM medially toward the tympanic space, producing a concave lateral surface of the TM, the most depressed part of which is called the *umbo* (Fig. 6). In the normal state, the TM is semitranslucent and affords a view of a portion of the ossicular chain and middle ear space through the EAC (Fig. 6).

Middle Ear Space

The middle ear space, or *tympanic space*, is commonly compartmentalized into the mesotympanum, epitympanum, and hypotympanum (Fig. 7). The *mesotympanum* is the portion immediately deep to the TM. It contains the *manubrium* of the *malleus*, long process and *lenticular process* of the incus, the stapes, tensor tympani, and stapes tendons, and the chorda tympani nerve (Fig. 7). The portion of the middle ear space above the roof of the EAC is the *epitympanum*, or *attic*, and contains the head of the malleus and body/short process of the incus. The epitympanum communicates with the mastoid antrum by way of a narrow passage, the *aditus ad antrum*. The *hypotympanum* is the portion of the middle ear below the floor of the EAC and contains the opening of the Eustachian tube anteriorly.

The tympanic space can be considered a six-walled chamber. The superior wall (*tegmen tympani*) or roof of the epitympanum is a thin layer of bone that separates the epitympanum and mastoid antrum from the middle cranial fossa.

The medial wall of the tympanic space separates the middle ear from the adjacent labyrinthine structures and includes several important bony landmarks (superior to inferior): the lateral *semicircular canal*, tympanic segment of the *facial nerve canal*, *oval window*, *cochlear promontory*, and *round window niche* (Figs. 7,8). The cochlear promontory, formed by the basal turn of the cochlear, is lodged between the oval and round windows. Its surface is grooved to accommodate the branches of the tympanic plexus (*Jacobson's nerve*), which enters the temporal bone through the *tympanic canaliculus*, just anterior to the jugular foramen. The posterior wall separates the middle ear from the mastoid air cells, except

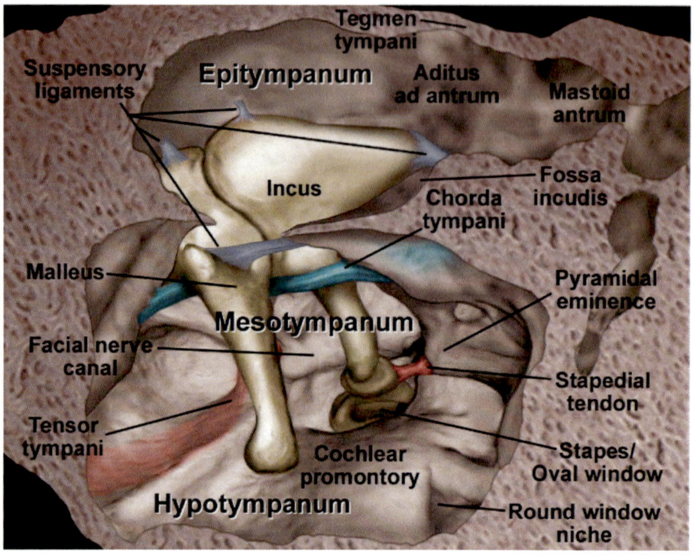

Fig. 7 The middle ear. 3D reconstruction of the microMR dataset. The outer surface of the temporal bone including the bony external auditory canal (EAC) has been removed. Note the attic or epitympanum in continuity with the mastoid antrum posteriorly. The mesotympanum is demarcated by the roof and floor of the EAC. The hypotympanum occupies that space inferior to the floor of the EAC. Suspensory ligaments of the ossicles are the illustrator's additions to the original reconstructions. Note the course of the chorda tympani nerve between the long process of the incus and manubrium of the malleus. Note the muscles of the middle ear to include the stapedial muscle and tendon emanating from the pyramidal eminence and its attachment to the neck of the stapes and the course of the tensor tympani muscle within its bony semi canal. Note the view of the *medial wall* of the tympanic cavity including the facial nerve canal, stapes at the level of the oval window, cochlear promontory, and round window niche

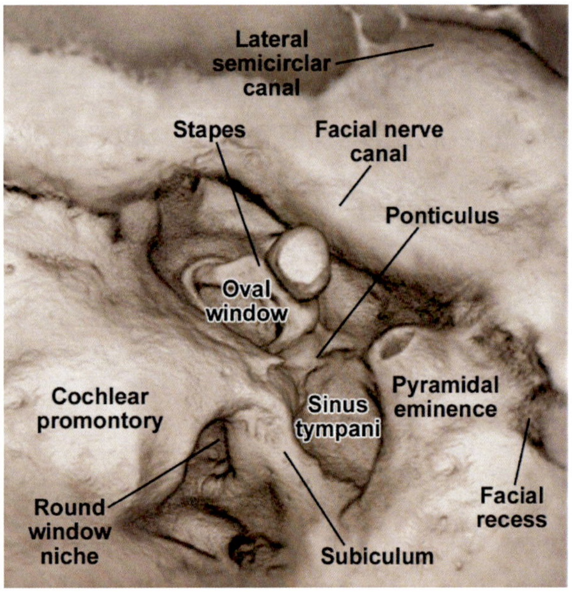

Fig. 8 The posteromedial wall of the middle ear. 3D reconstruction of the microCT dataset. Note the pyramidal eminence projecting from the posterior wall of the middle ear. Its hollow orifice transmits the stapial tendon. Deep to the eminence is the sinus tympani, a recess separated from the round window niche inferiorly by a bony ridge, the subiculum, and from the oval window niche anterosuperiorly by another bony ridge, the ponticulus. The facial recess is found lateral to the pyramidal eminence. The lateral semicircular canal creates a bony overhang superior to the oval window along the medial wall of the middle ear. Coursing beneath the lateral canal is the tympanic segment of the facial nerve canal. Note the cochlear promontory and round window niche inferior and posterior to the oval window

along its deficient superior margin, where it permits communication between the *attic* and the *mastoid antrum*. It presents several notable features (superior to inferior): the *fossa incudis* (a small recess that receives the short process of the incus), the *pyramidal eminence* (PE), which transmits the *stapedial tendon*, and two additional recesses on either side of the PE, the *sinus tympani* medially and the *facial recess* laterally (Figs. 7, 8). The sinus tympani is separated from the oval window by an anterior bony ridge, the *ponticulus*, and from the round window niche by an inferior bony ridge, the *subiculum* (Fig. 8). Pars tensa cholesteatomas will commonly extend along the posterior wall to involve the sinus tympani. The PE will often obscure this recess at the time of surgical tympanomastoid exposure. Therefore, it is important to evaluate this recess with CT preoperatively to exclude occult extension of disease.

The lateral wall of the middle ear is primarily composed of the TM and the incomplete tympanic ring of bone to which the membrane is attached (Fig. 9). As was mentioned previously, the tympanic ring is deficient superiorly (Notch of Rivinus), resulting in the laxity of the membrane adjacent to the notch (*pars flaccida*). The confluence of the lateral wall of the middle ear and the roof of the EAC form a sharp spur of bone, known as the *scutum*. Deep to the pars flaccida is a small recess, *Prussak's space*, bordered superiorly and laterally by the *scutum*, and medially by the neck of the malleus, which is a common site for pars flaccida cholesteatoma.

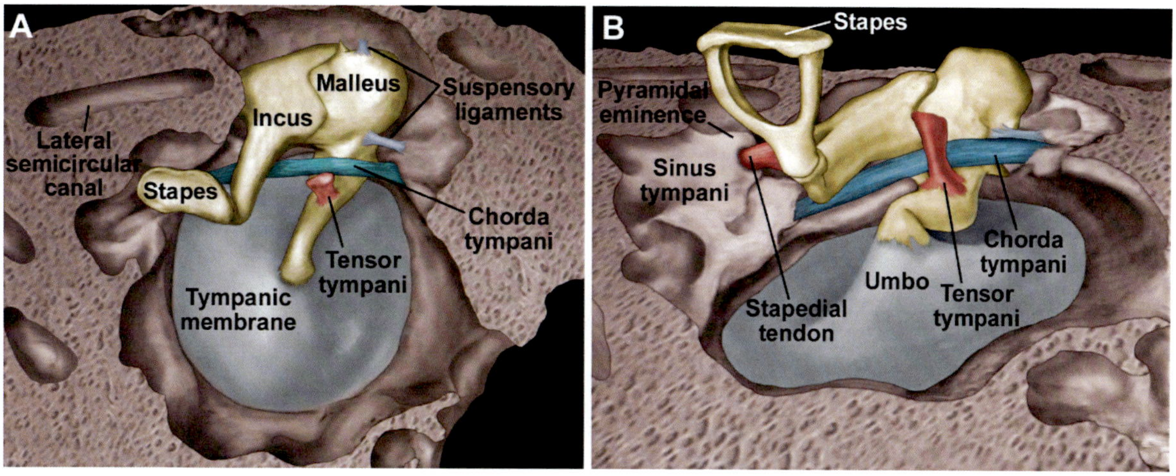

Fig. 9 The lateral wall of the middle ear. (**a**) 3D reconstruction of the microMR dataset. Note the inner surface of the tympanic membrane, the course of the chorda tympani nerve and the cut edge of the tensor tympani muscle proximal to its attachment to the medial surface of the manubrium of the malleus. (**b**) Inferior oblique view of the lateral wall to include a view of the posterior wall demonstrates the pyramidal eminence transmitting the stapedial tendon that attaches to the neck of the stapes. Note the posterior recess medial to the pyramidal eminence, the sinus tympani

Close to the bony ring are the two apertures (posterior and anterior) that transmit the *chorda tympani nerve* into and out of the middle ear space (Fig. 9). The anterior wall separates the middle ear from the adjacent carotid canal. The *Eustachian tube* and *semi canal of the tensor tympani* openings are found along its ventral extent. The inferior wall or floor is narrow and consists of a thin plate of bone that separates the middle ear from the *jugular fossa*. Occasionally, this bone may be dehiscent, with the jugular vein being visible through theTM.

The Auditory Ossicles

The ossicular chain is responsible for the transmission of sound-induced vibrations of the TM to the oval window. The chain is composed of three bones: the *malleus*, *incus*, and *stapes*, which are named after the (once) common objects they resemble (hammer, anvil, and stirrup) (Figs. 10–13). The malleus consists of a round head, short neck, two small processes (anterior and lateral), and an elongated handle or *manubrium*. The manubrium of the malleus is attached to the TM. The head of the malleus articulates with the body of the incus within the epitympanum or attic. This articulation is therefore not visible on routine otoscopy. The malleus and incus share a saddle-shaped diarthrodial joint at their articulation in the epitympanum. The incus consists of a trapezoidal body, short and long crura or processes, and a rounded *lenticular process*, projecting medially from the long process, which articulates with the head of the stapes. The stapes consists of a round head, short neck, anterior and posterior crura, and an oval footplate. The ossicles are stabilized by numerous *suspensory ligaments* (Figs. 7, 9), joint capsules, and two tendons: the *tensor tympani tendon*, which attaches to the upper part of the manubrium of the malleus, and the *stapedial tendon*, which attaches to the neck of the stapes. The incus has the least number of stabilizers and is therefore most commonly dislocated with middle ear trauma. The footplate of the stapes is fixed to the edges of the oval window by the *annular ligament*. Vibration of the footplate initiates the displacement of fluid within the vestibule of the inner ear (Fig. 14), which ultimately leads to the stimulation of the hair cells within the cochlea, resulting in a transfer of mechanical energy to electrical energy conducted by way of the cochlear nerve to the brainstem.

The Inner Ear

The *labyrinth* is a system of membranous sacs and ducts filled with *endolymph*, surrounded by *perilymph*,

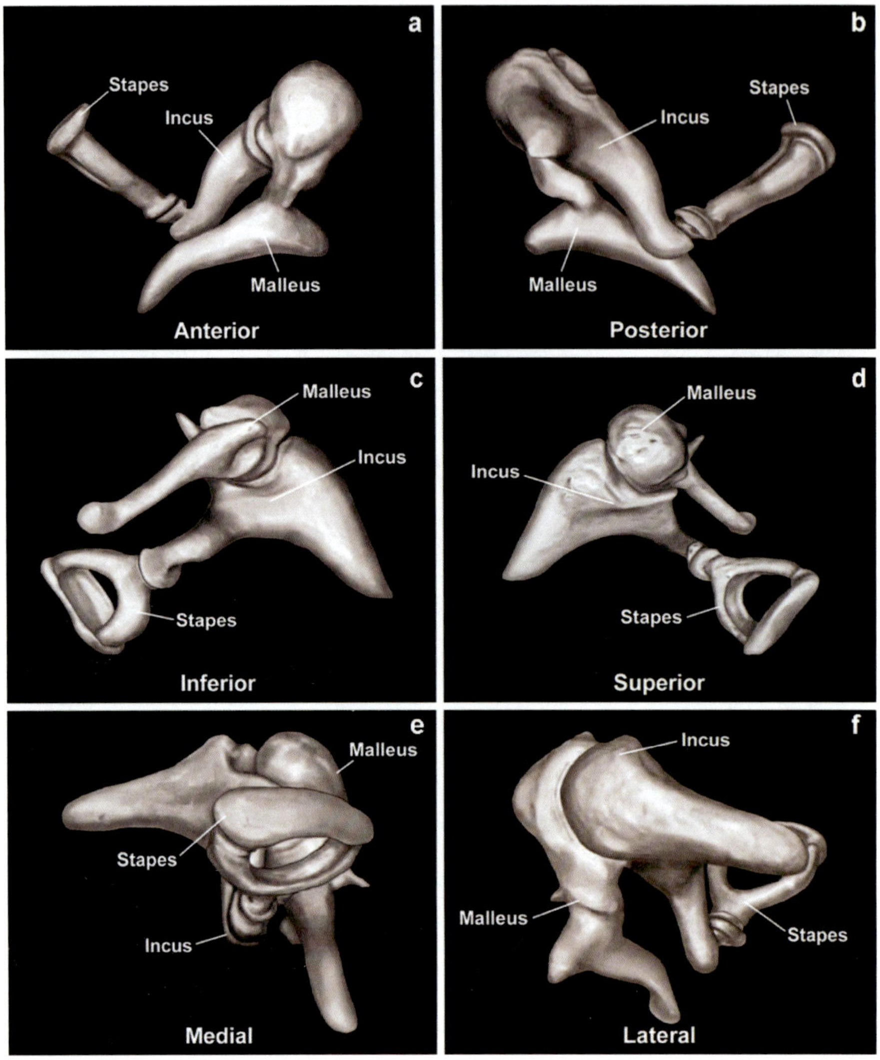

Fig. 10 The middle ear ossicles. 3D reconstruction of the microCT dataset. (**a**) Anterior and (**b**) posterior views of the ossicular chain. Note the oblique orientation of the malleus and incus angled superolaterally to inferomedially and the superior angulation of the stapes. (**c**) Inferior and (**d**) superior views of the ossicular chain. Note the oblique orientation of the malleus and incus angled anterolaterally to posteromedially and the slightly posterior angulation of the stapes. (**e**) Medial and (**f**), lateral views of the ossicular chain. Note the posterior orientation of the short process of the incus and the superior angulation of the stapes

and encased in bone (*otic capsule*) (Figs. 15–20). The auditory component (*cochlea*) occupies the anterior portion of the labyrinth and is shaped like a conch schell. Its lumen consists of 2.5 radial turns (basal, middle, and apical) around a cribriform bony column, the *modiolus*, which transmits the fibers of the *cochlear nerve*. The vestibular apparatus is housed posteriorly in the *vestibule* and *semicircular canals*. These structures are embedded within the otic capsule to which the membranes are fixed at given points.

The endolymphatic compartment of the membranous labyrinth consists of the *cochlear duct* (*scala media*), *saccule*, *utricle*, *semicircular ducts* (superior, lateral, and posterior), and the *endolymphatic duct* transmitted by the *vestibular aqueduct* to its confluence with the endolymphatic sac found beneath the dura along the posterior surface of the petrous portion of the temporal bone (Fig. 3). The *cochlear duct* occupies the scala media within the lumen of the cochlea and is attached to the outer walls of the cochlear turns. The basilar end of the cochlear duct extends along the floor of the vestibule and communicates with the saccule by way of the short *ductus reuniens*. Within the bony vestibule, the *saccule* is attached to the medial wall of the vestibule wherein lies the vertically oriented *saccular macula*, the neurosensorial epithelium that acts in concert with the horizontally oriented *utricular macula* to detect linear acceleration. The *utricle* is fixed to the anteromedial wall of the vestibule where the *utricular macula* has its origin, extending posteriorly along the floor

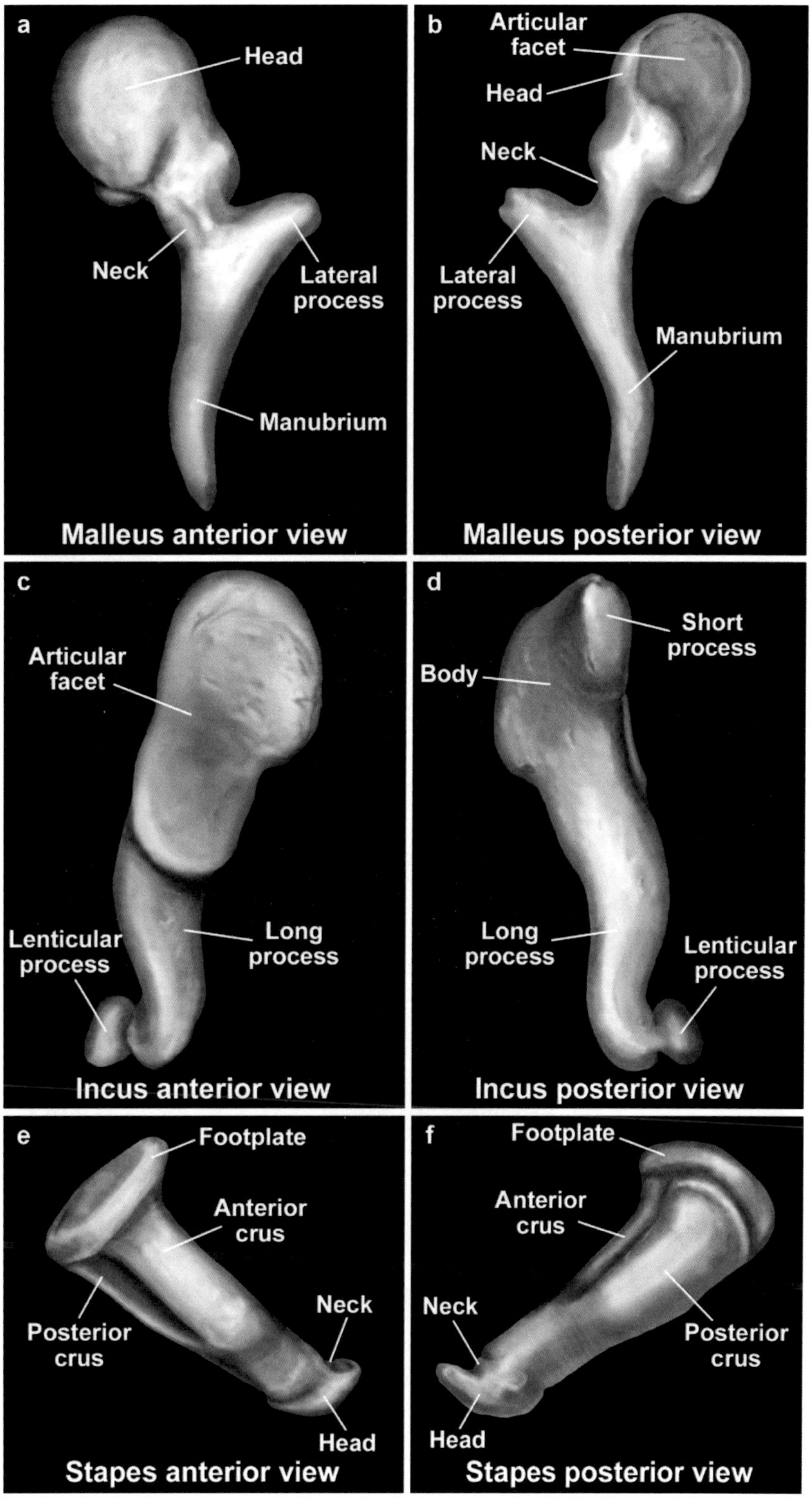

Fig. 11 Anterior–posterior perspectives of the disarticulated ossicles. 3D reconstructions of the microCT dataset. (**a**) Anterior and (**b**) posterior views of the malleus demonstrating head, neck, lateral process, and manubrium. Note the articular facet of the mallear head on the posterior view. (**c**) Anterior and (**d**) posterior views of the incus demonstrating body, short and long processes, and the lenticular process. Note the articular facet of the incus occupying the anterior surface of the body. (**e**) Anterior and (**f**) posterior views of the stapes demonstrating the head, neck, anterior and posterior crura, and the footplate

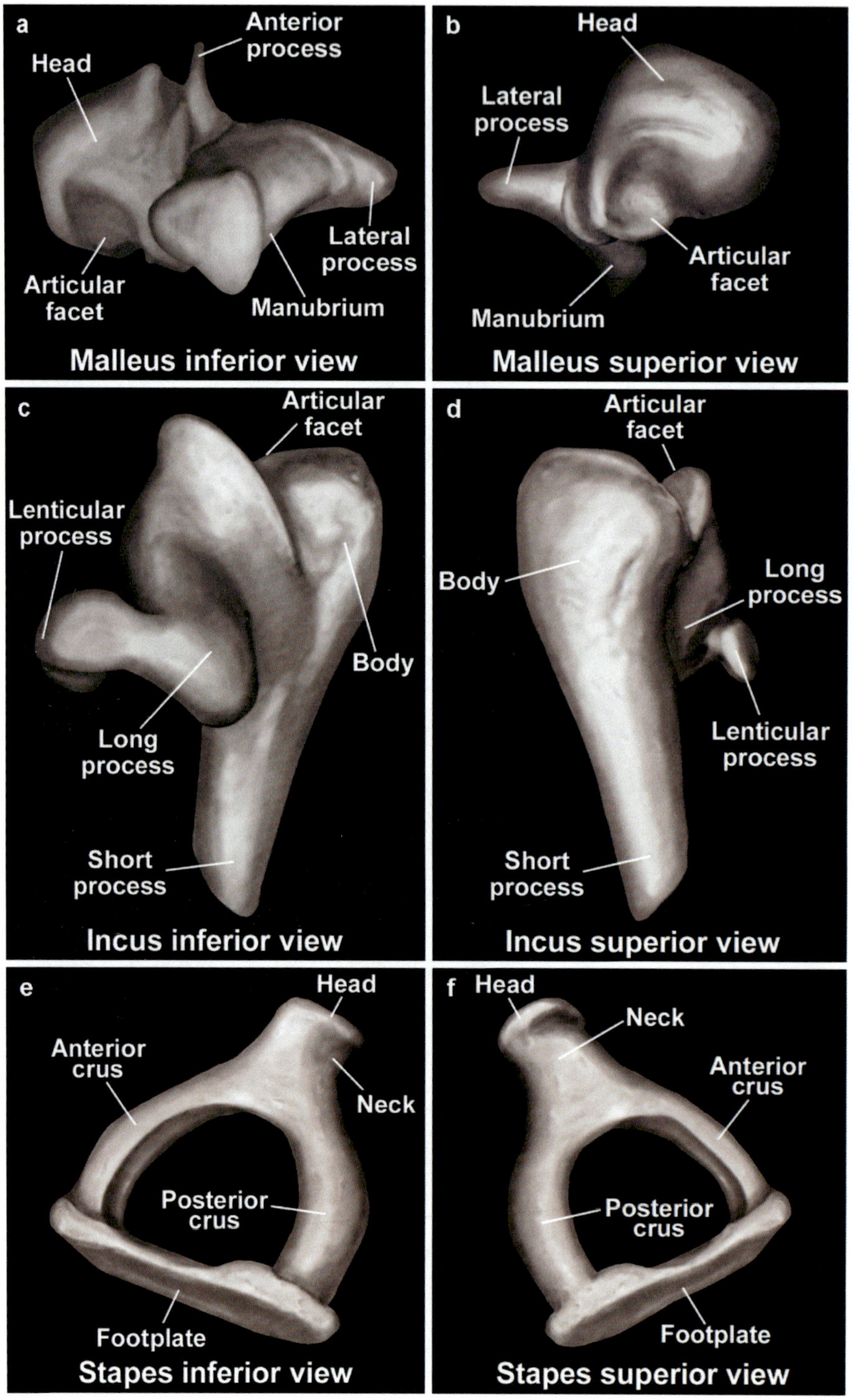

Fig. 12 Superior–inferior perspectives of the disarticulated ossicles. 3D reconstructions of the microCT dataset. (**a**) Inferior and (**b**) superior views of the malleus demonstrating the head, neck, lateral process, anterior process, and manubrium. Note the articular facet of the mallear head. (**c**) Superior and (**d**) inferior views of the incus demonstrating the body, short and long processes, and the lenticular process. Note the medial orientation of the lenticular process that articulates with the head of the stapes. (**e**) Superior and (**f**) inferior views of the stapes demonstrating the head, neck, anterior and posterior crura, and the footplate. Note that the posterior crus is slightly thicker and has less curvature than the anterior crus

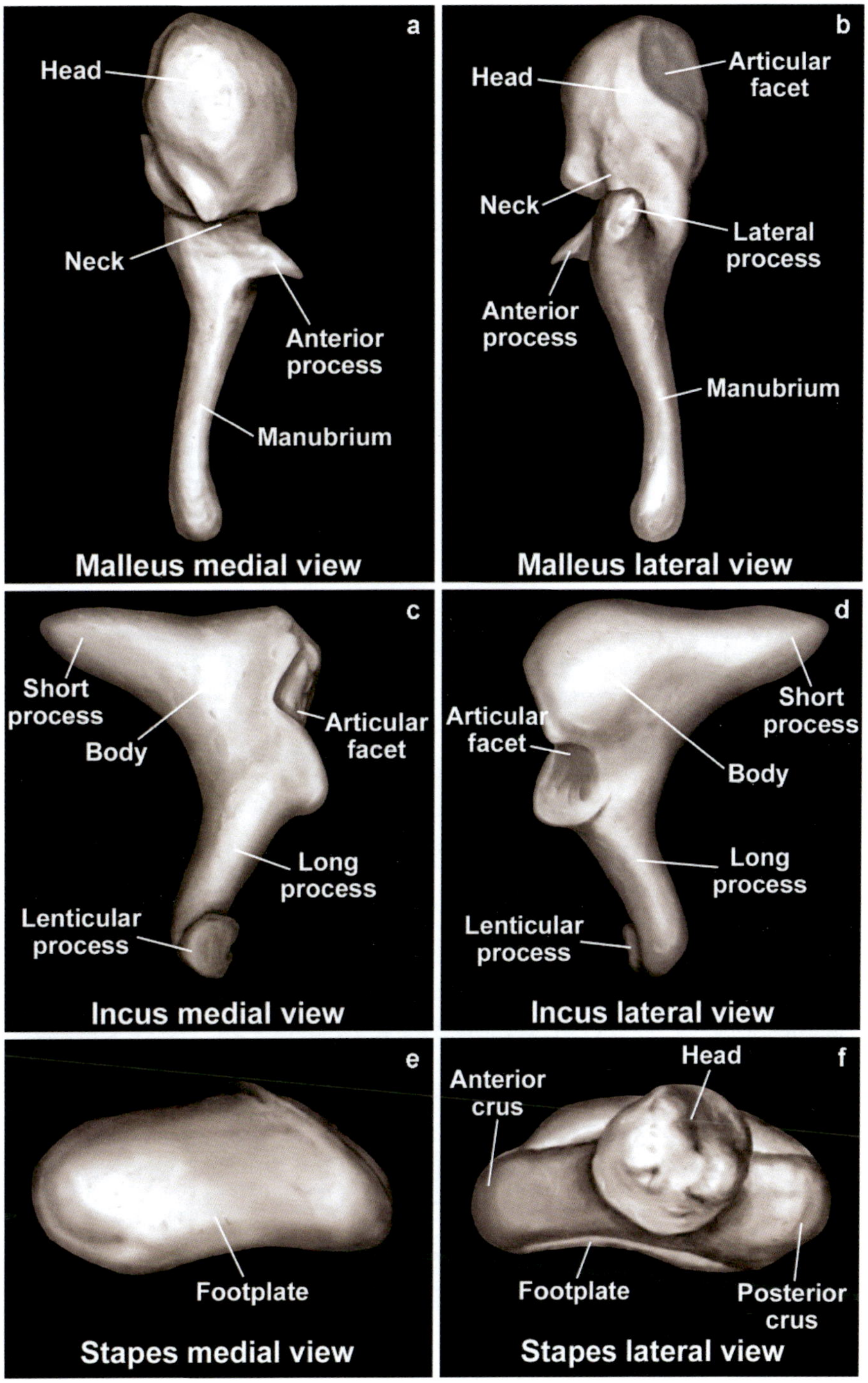

Fig. 13 Medial–lateral perspectives of the disarticulated ossicles. 3D reconstructions of the microCT dataset. (**a**) Medial and (**b**) lateral views of the malleus demonstrating the head, neck, lateral process, anterior process, and manubrium. Note the articular facet of the mallear head on the lateral view. (**c**) Medial and (**d**) lateral views of the incus demonstrating the body, short and long processes, and the lenticular process. Note the articular facet of incus, the posteriorly oriented short process, and the articular surface of the lenticular process. (**e**) Medial and (**f**) lateral views of the stapes demonstrating the head, neck, anterior and posterior crura, and the footplate. The footplate is convex superiorly and concave inferiorly

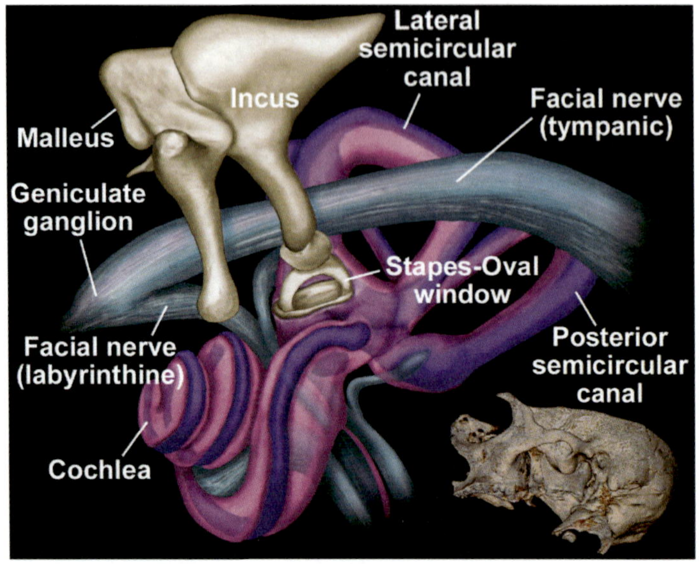

Fig. 14 Relationship between the ossicles and the inner ear. 3D reconstruction from the microMR dataset in a steep inferior anterolateral oblique projection (*inset*). Note the position of the footplate of the stapes at the level of the oval window. The perilymphatic space is segmented in *pink*, and the endolymphatic structures in *purple*. Note the relationship between the tympanic segment of the facial nerve and the lateral semicircular canal and oval window

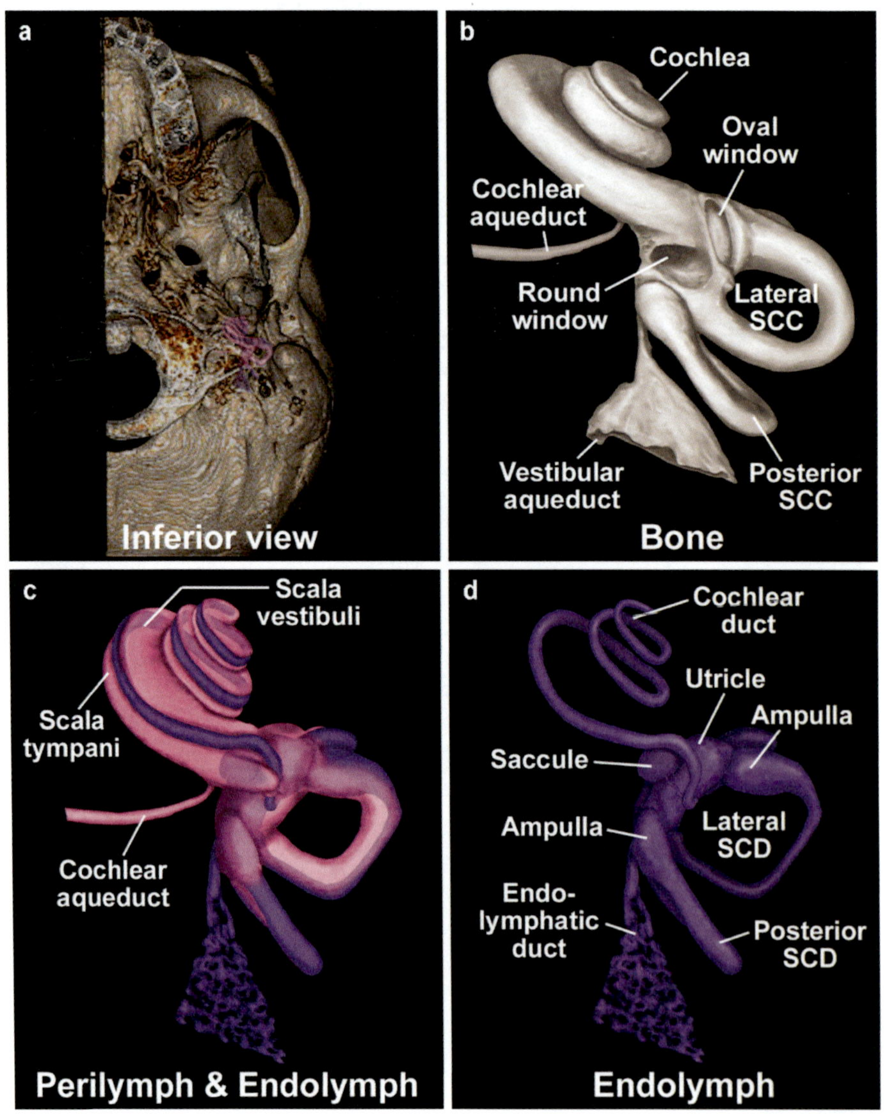

Fig. 15 The inner ear. Inferior views of 3D reconstructions from microscopy datasets. (**a**) 3D MDCT reference image with superimposed labyrinth. (**b**) MicroCT reconstruction of the bony labyrinth. (**c**) MicroMR reconstruction of the membranous labyrinth to include perilymphatic and endolymphatic spaces. (**d**) MicroMR reconstruction of the endolymphatic structures of the membranous labyrinth only. Note that the semicircular ducts (endolymph) are attached to the outer wall of the canals and occupy about one-fourth of the volume of their respective canals, the remainder being perilymphatic space

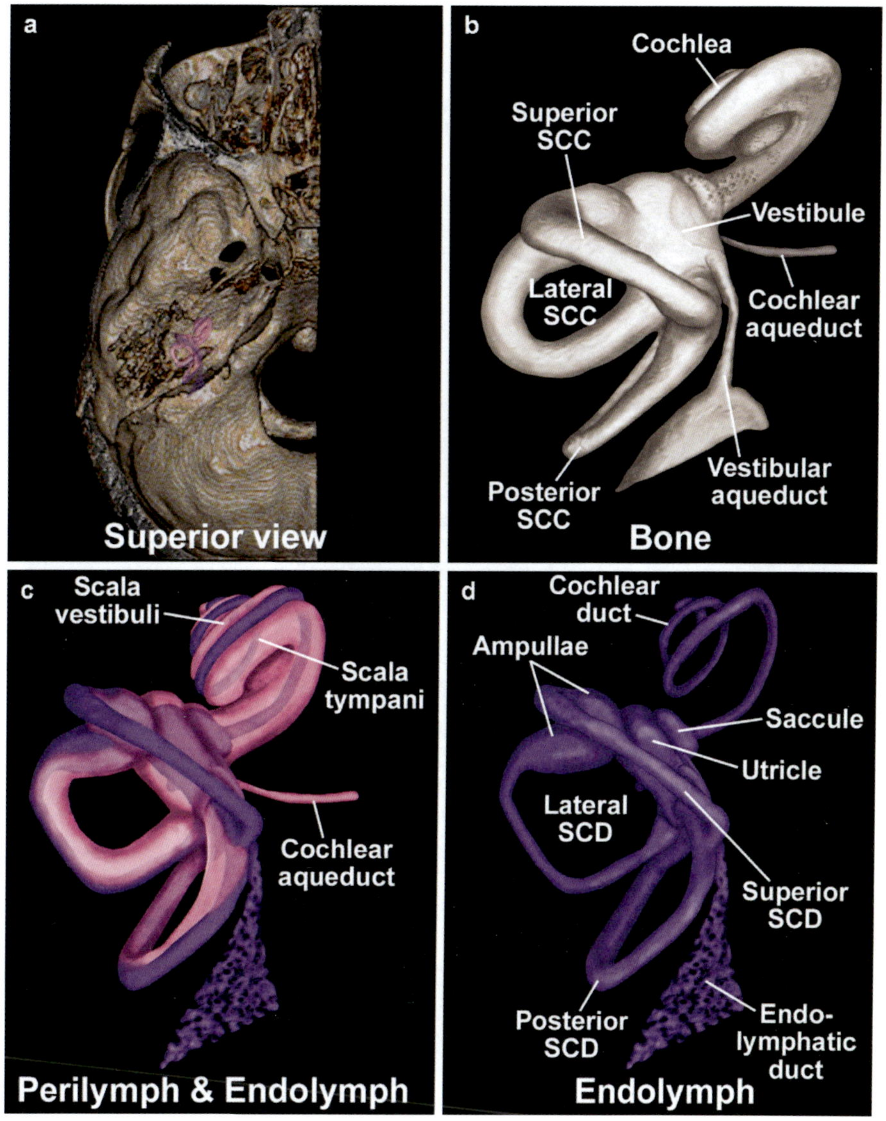

Fig. 16 The inner ear. Superior views of 3D reconstructions from microscopy datasets. (**a**) 3D MDCT reference image with superimposed labyrinth. (**b**) MicroCT reconstruction of the bony labyrinth. (**c**) MicroMR reconstruction of the membranous labyrinth to include perilymphatic and endolymphatic spaces. (**d**) MicroMR reconstruction of the endolymphatic structures of the membranous labyrinth only. Note the vestibular aqueduct arising from the medial wall of the vestibule posteriorly

of the utricle. The utricle lies within the *elliptical recess*, an ellipsoid depression in the anterosuperior aspect of the medial wall of the vestibule. The saccule lies inferior to the utricle within a rounded depression along the anteroinferior aspect of the medial wall of the vestibule (*spherical recess*). These recesses are separated by a bony ridge, the *vestibular crest* (Fig. 21). The lateral wall of the vestibule is notable for the openings of the *oval window*, and both limbs of the lateral semicircular canal (Fig. 22). The roof of the vestibule receives the ampullated limb of the superior semicircular canal and more posteriorly the *common crus*, the fused nonampullated ends of the superior and posterior canals (Figs. 21, 22). The ampullated end of the posterior semicircular canal opens up into the inferior aspect of the posterior wall of the vestibule (Fig. 22). The opening of the scala vestibuli of the cochlea is located along the floor of the vestibule just inferior and anterior to the oval window (Fig. 22).

The endolymphatic *semicircular ducts* (superior, lateral and posterior) are attached to the outer walls of their respective canals (Figs. 15–20). They each have an ampullated end, which contains the *crista ampullaris*, the neuroepithelial sensory organ that detects angular or rotational acceleration. They define three planes of rotation: a horizontal plane defined by the

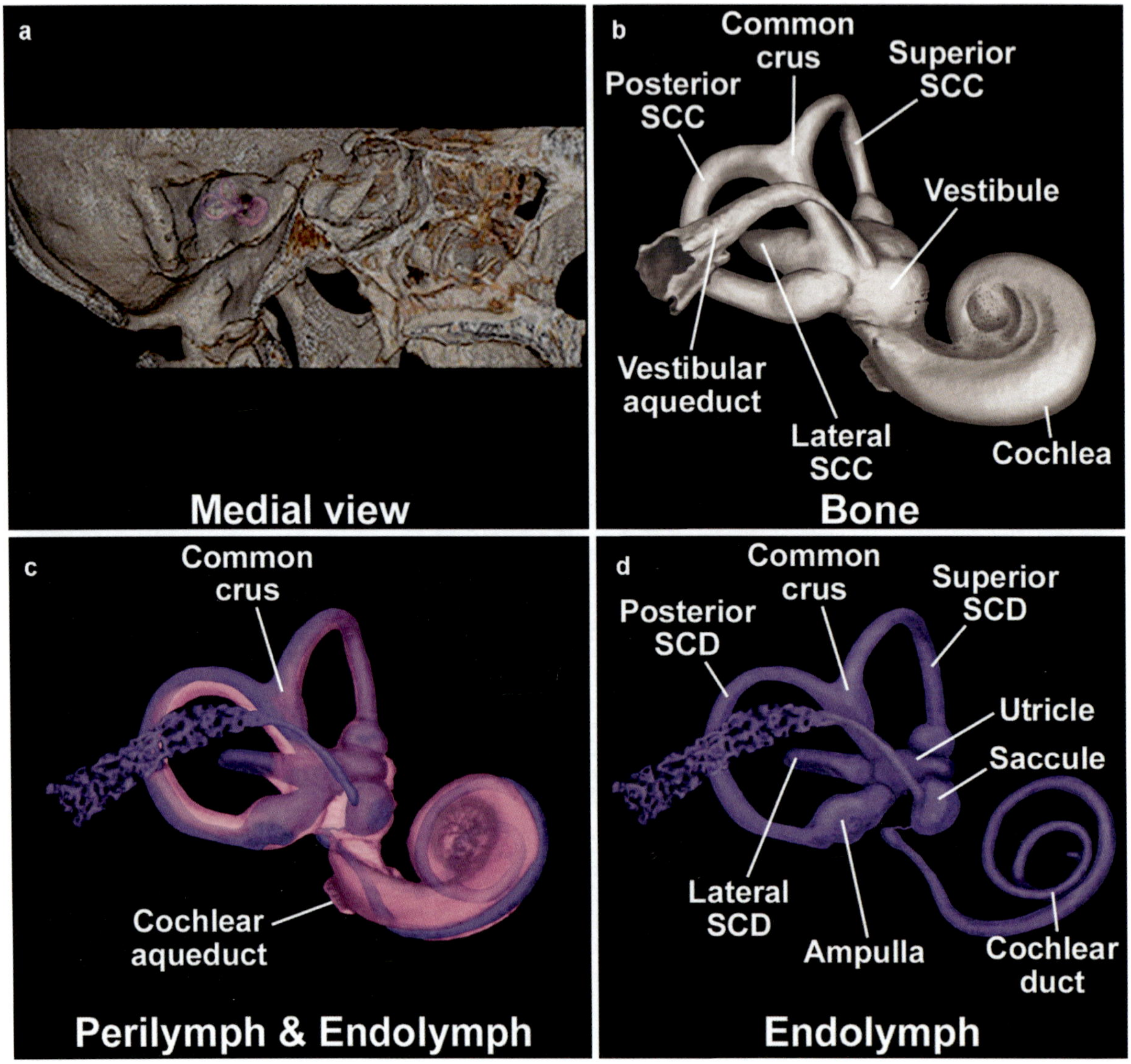

Fig. 17 The inner ear. Medial views of 3D reconstructions from microscopy datasets. (**a**) 3D MDCT reference image with superimposed labyrinth. (**b**) MicroCT reconstruction of the bony labyrinth. (**c**) MicroMR reconstruction of the membranous labyrinth to include perilymphatic and endolymphatic spaces. (**d**) MicroMR reconstruction of the endolymphatic structures of the membranous labyrinth only. Note the relationship between the ellipsoidal utricle superiorly and the spherical saccule inferiorly within the vestibule. Also note that the vestibular aqueduct opens into the posteromedial wall of the vestibule just anterior to the opening of the common crus. The endolymphatic duct arises from the posterior wall of the saccule, is joined by the short utriculosaccular duct (not shown) coming from the utricle, and exits the vestibule by way of the vestibular aqueduct

paired lateral canals, and two pairs of oblique vertical planes, oriented at 90° to each other, defined by the ipsilateral superior and the contralateral posterior ducts. The semicircular ducts occupy approximately one-fourth of the volume of their respective canals. Both nonampullated ends of the superior and posterior ducts (and canals) are fused, forming the *common crus*. The semicircular ducts each communicate with the utricle within the upper portion of the vestibule. The *endolymphatic duct* (Figs. 15–20) arises from the posterior wall of the saccule, communicates with the utricle by way of the short *utriculosaccular duct*, and exits the vestibule through a small opening just anterior and inferior to the opening of the common crus

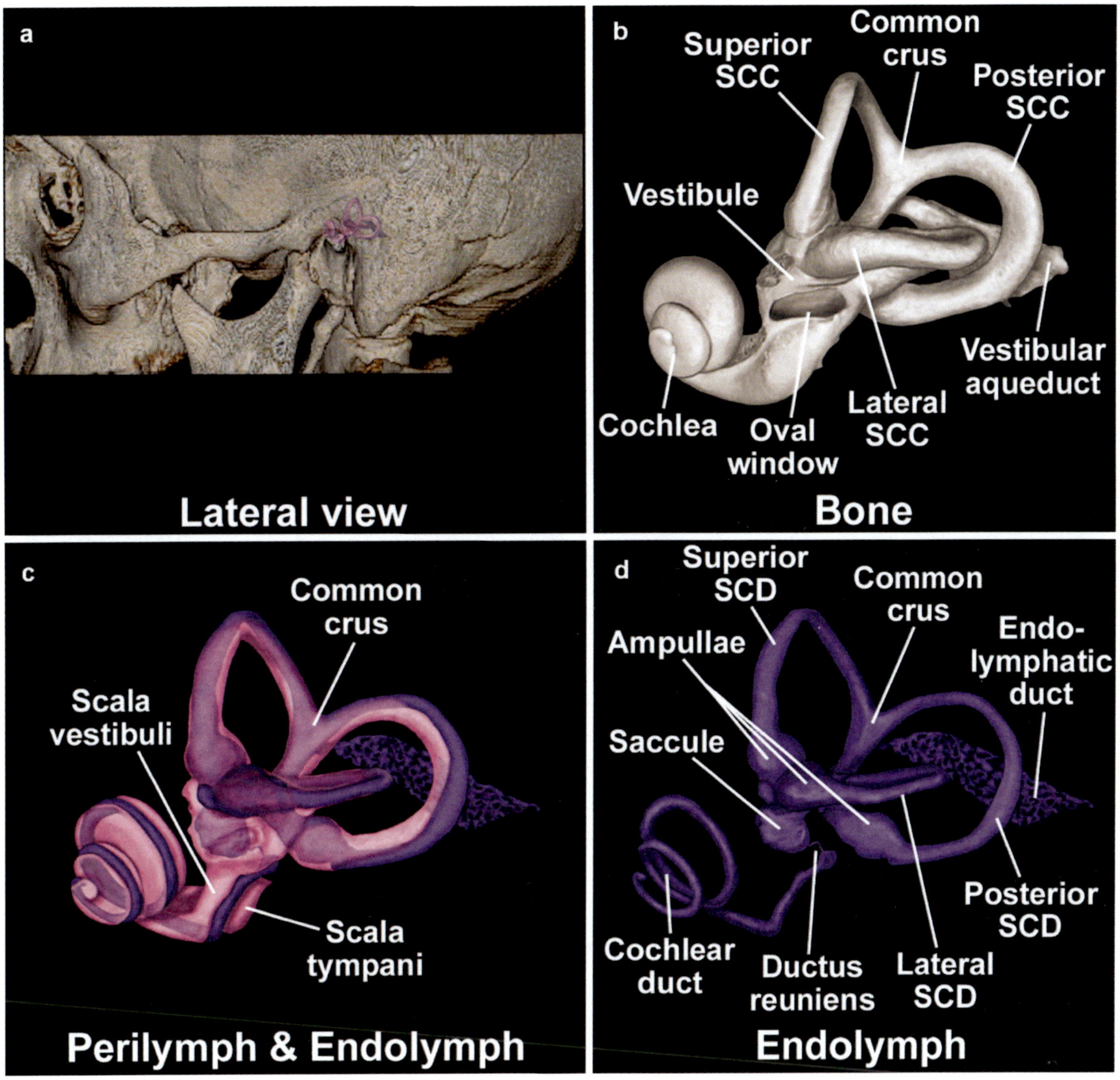

Fig. 18 The inner ear. Lateral views of 3D reconstructions from microscopy datasets. (**a**) 3D MDCT reference image with superimposed labyrinth. (**b**) MicroCT reconstruction of the bony labyrinth. (**c**) MicroMR reconstruction of the membranous labyrinth to include the perilymphatic and endolymphatic spaces. (**d**) MicroMR reconstruction of the endolymphatic structures of the membranous labyrinth only. Note the fusion of the nonampullated ends of the superior and posterior semicircular canals and ducts to form the common crus. Also note the extension of the cochlear duct out of the basal turn of the cochlea along the floor of the vestibule and its connection to the saccule by way of the ductus reuniens. Third, note the proximity of the ampullae of the superior and lateral semicircular ducts

along the posterior superior aspect of the medial wall of the vestibule (Fig. 21). It is transmitted through the petrous portion of the temporal bone by way of the *vestibular aqueduct* and terminates in the endolymphatic sac (Fig. 22). Thus, the common crus serves as a landmark for identifying the location of the proximal segment of the vestibular aqueduct.

The perilymphatic compartment fills that portion of the labyrinth not occupied by the endolymphatic structures (Figs. 15–20). It is similar in composition to the subarachnoid spaces of the central nervous system with which it may potentially communicate by way of the cochlear aqueduct (Fig. 2). The reported patency of the cochlear aqueduct varies, one study demonstrating

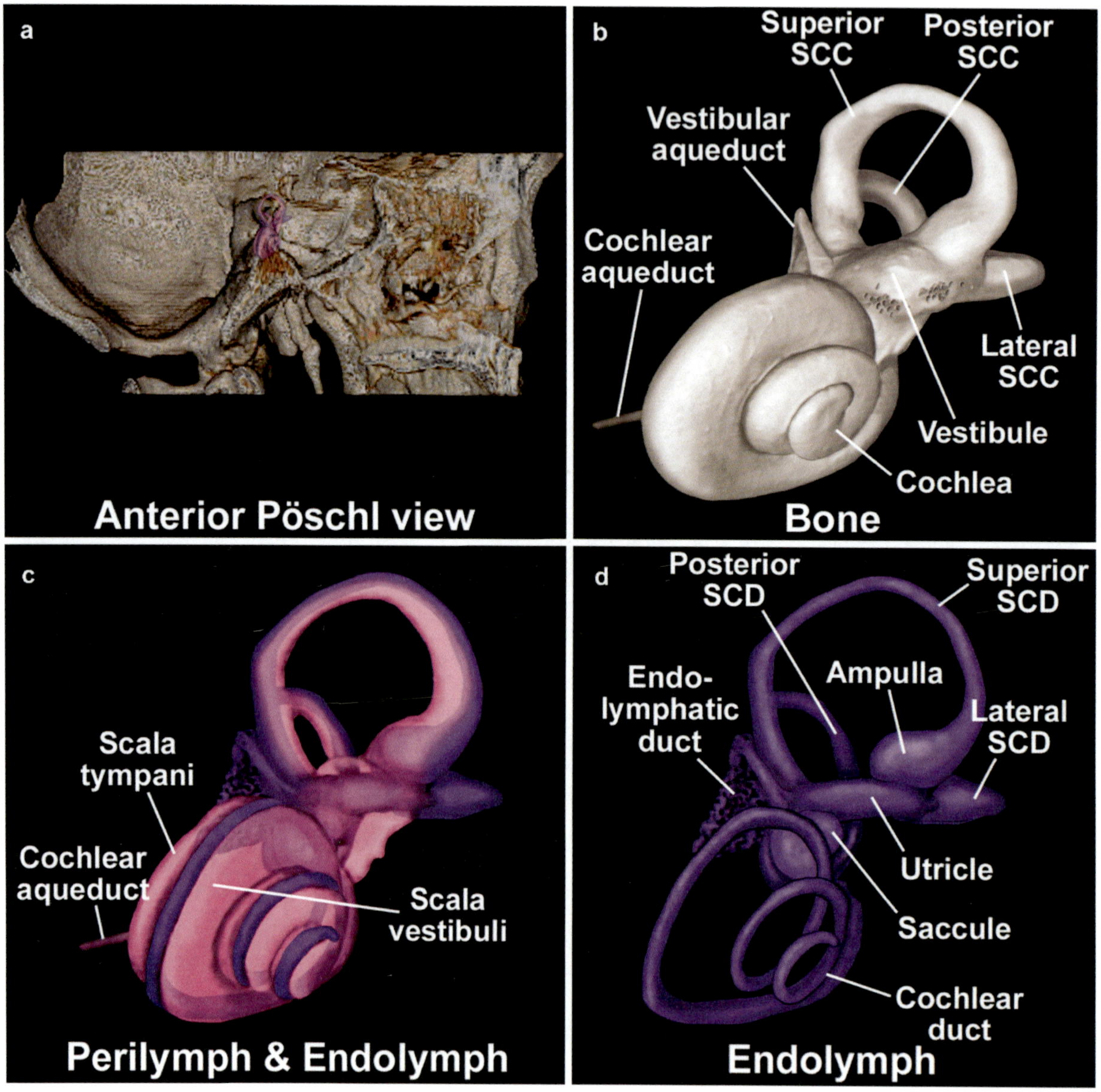

Fig. 19 The inner ear. Right anterior oblique (anterior Pöschl projection) views of 3D reconstructions from microscopy datasets. (**a**) 3D MDCT reference image with superimposed labyrinth. (**b**) MicroCT reconstruction of the bony labyrinth. (**c**) MicroMR reconstruction of the membranous labyrinth to include the perilymphatic and endolymphatic spaces. (**d**) MicroMR reconstruction of the endolymphatic structures of the membranous labyrinth only. Note the relationship between the ellipsoidal utricle superiorly and the spherical saccule inferomedially within the vestibule. Also note the anterior position of the scala vestibuli and the posterior position of the scala tympani within the cochlea

patency in only 34% of normal postmortem exams [1]. There are two perilympatic compartments within the cochlea; the *scala vestibuli*, which opens into the floor of the vestibule and conducts the fluid wave produced at the oval window, and the *scala tympani*, which communicates with the scala vestibuli through a small defect at the cochlear apex (the *helicotrema*) and ends at the *round window* membrane. Perilymphatic fluid displacement at the *oval window* is accommodated by the perilymphatic fluid displacement at the *round window* membrane. The two perilymphatic scala of the cochlea are separated by a partial bony partition, the *spiral lamina*, which extends outward from the modiolus of the cochlea. The partition is further extended to

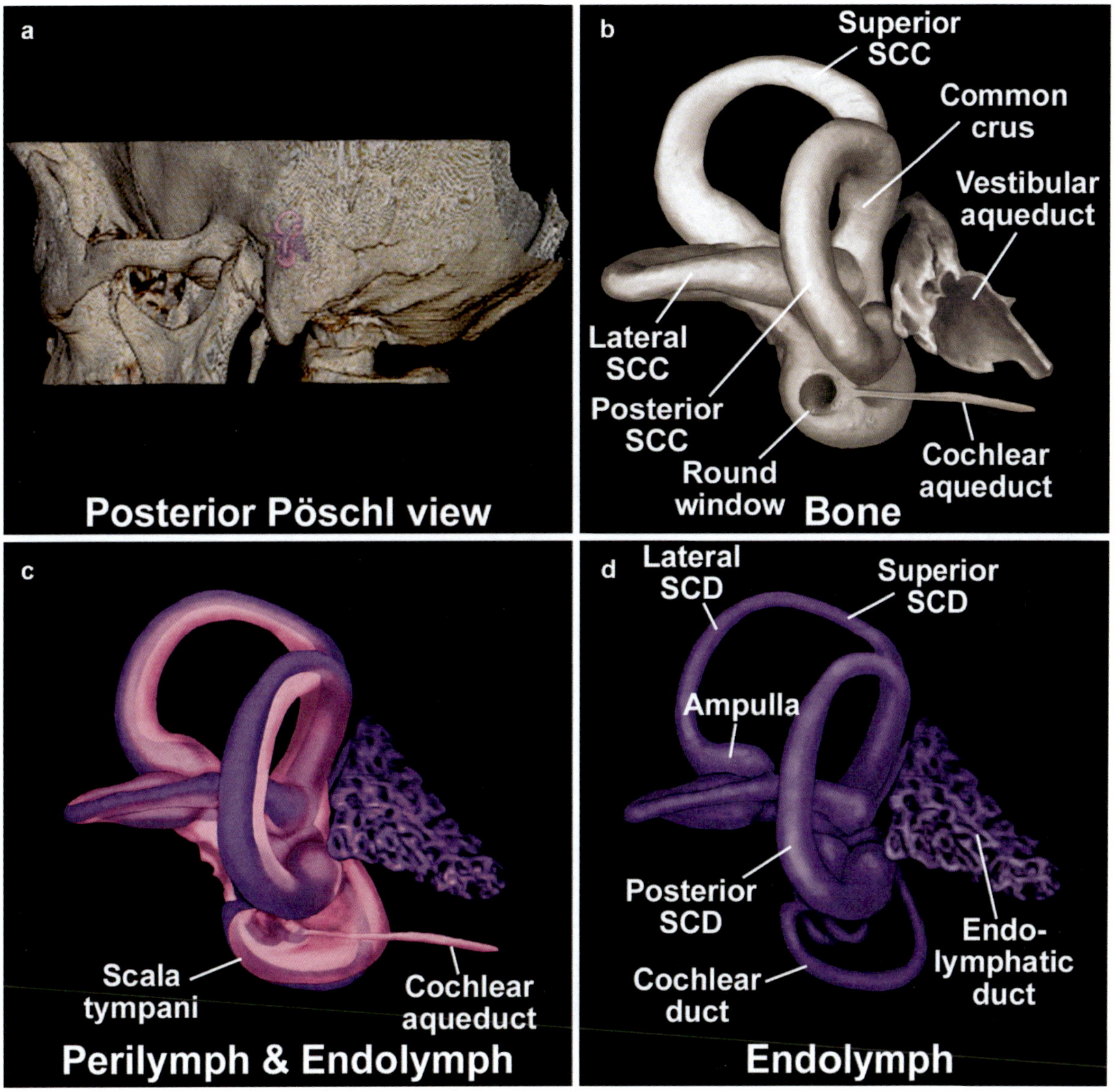

Fig. 20 The inner ear. Left posterior oblique (posterior Pöschl projection) views of 3D reconstructions from microscopy datasets. (**a**) 3D MDCT reference image with superimposed labyrinth. (**b**) MicroCT reconstruction of the bony labyrinth. (**c**) MicroMR reconstruction of the membranous labyrinth to include the perilymphatic and endolymphatic spaces. (**d**) MicroMR reconstruction of the endolymphatic structures of the membranous labyrinth only. Note the cochlear aqueduct opening into the scala tympani of the cochlea just inside the round window. Also note the location of the vestibular aqueduct medial to the common crus

the outer wall of the cochlea by way of the *basilar membrane*. The modiolus is anchored to the surrounding otic capsule by the *interscalar septa*, complete bony partitions that separate the cochlear turns. The previously mentioned endolymphatic cochlear duct (scala media), distributed along the outer wall of the cochlear lumen, is separated from the scala vestibuli by a thin membrane (*Reissner's membrane*) and from the scala tympani by the more substantial basilar membrane. Perilymph fills much of the lateral aspect of the vestibule and approximately three-fourths of the volume of the semicircular canals.

Innervation of the neurosensory epithelium of the inner ear is by way of the VIIIth cranial nerve, or

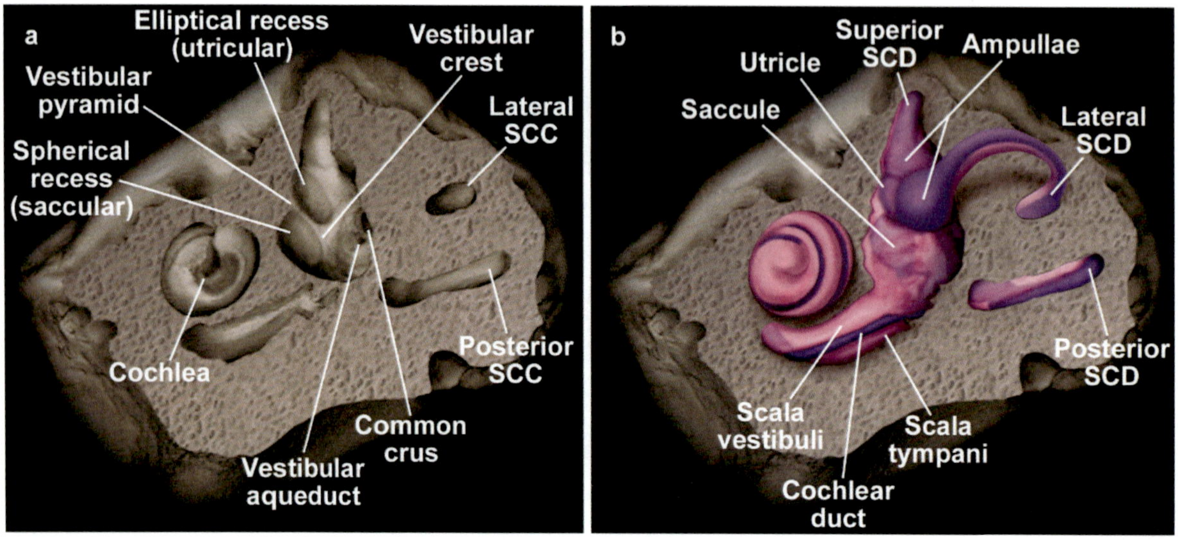

Fig. 21 Medial wall of the labyrinth. (**a**) 3D reconstruction of the microCT dataset demonstrating the exposed medial wall of the bony labyrinth and (**b**) superimposed 3D reconstruction of the membranous labyrinth from the microMR dataset. Note the elliptical and spherical recesses accommodating the medal surfaces of the utricle and saccule respectively. They are separated by a bony ridge, the vestibular crest. The vestibular pyramid, a small projection of cribriform bone accommodating the superior vestibular nerve fibers innervating the utricular macula, is found at the superior edge of the vestibular crest. The ampullated end of the superior semicircular canal opens into the roof of the vestibule. Note the opening of the vestibular aqueduct anterior and inferior to the opening of the common crus

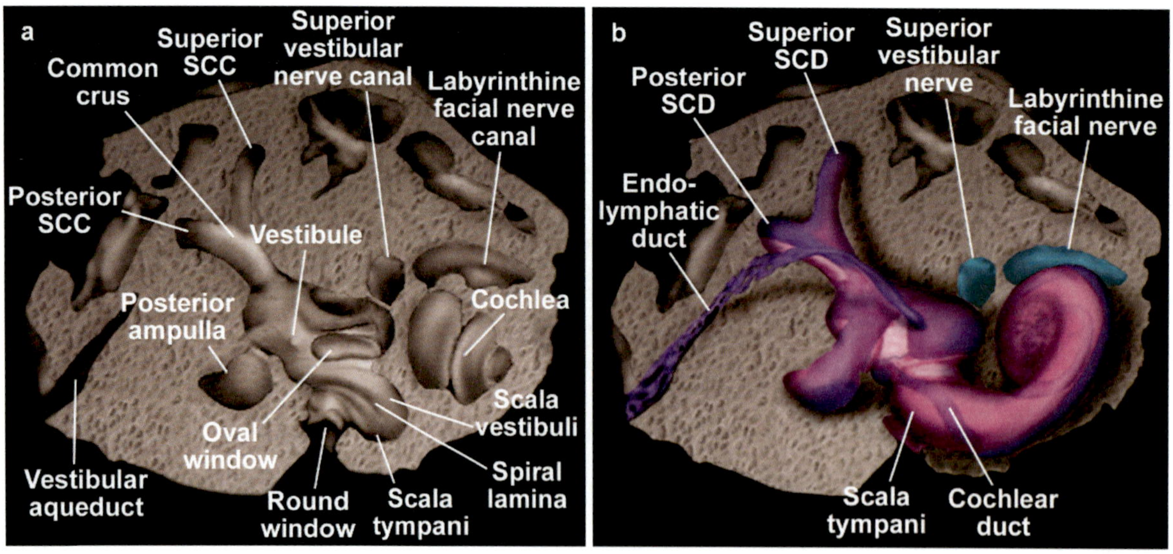

Fig. 22 Lateral wall of the labyrinth. (**a**) 3D reconstruction of the microCT dataset demonstrating the exposed lateral wall of the bony labyrinth and (**b**) superimposed 3D reconstruction of the membranous labyrinth from the microMR dataset. Note footplate of the stapes in the oval window. The spiral lamina is in continuity with the floor of the vestibule. The vestibule communicates with the scala vestibuli of the cochlea through a small oval-shaped aperture. Inferior to the spiral lamina, the scala tympani terminates at the round window. The ampullated end of the posterior semicircular canal opens into the posterior wall of the vestibule. Note the opening of the fused nonampullated ends of the superior and posterior semicircular canals, known as the common crus, along the posterior wall of the vestibule.

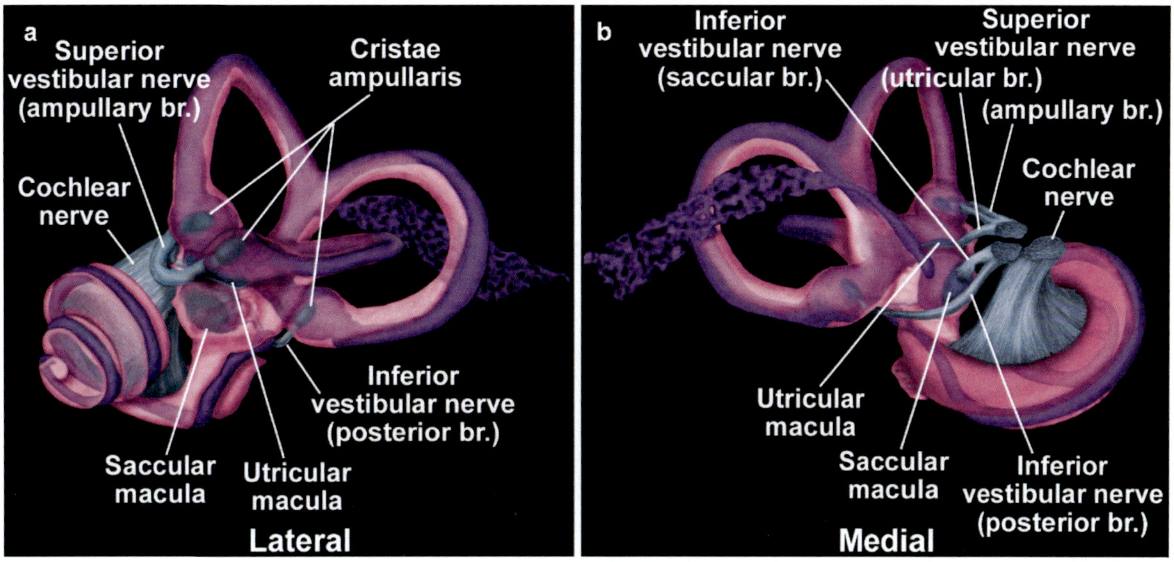

Fig. 23 Innervation of the inner ear. (**a**) Lateral and (**b**) medial views of the membranous labyrinth including nerve supply. 3D reconstructions from the microMR dataset. Intracanalicular nerve segments, avulsed during dissection, have been added to the original images. Superior and inferior vestibular nerves innervate the vestibular apparatus and the cochlear nerve innervates the auditory apparatus of the cochlea. Note that the superior vestibular nerve has an ampullary branch supplying the cristae ampullaris of the superior and lateral semicircular ducts and a utricular branch supplying the utricular macula. The inferior vestibular nerve has two branches, the saccular branch innervating the saccular macula, and the posterior branch, innervating the crista ampullaris of the posterior semicircular duct. The cochlear nerve is composed of efferent fibers from all the spiral ganglia cells found at the base of the spiral lamina. They arborize through multiple small channels within the modiolus and coalesce within the cochlear nerve aperture at the apex of the internal auditory canal (IAC). Spiral ganglia cell afferent fibers transmit input from the hair cells of the organ of Corti within the cochlear duct (scala media)

vestibulocochlear nerve, which enters the temporal bone through the IAC (Figs. 23–27). The *cochlear nerve*, a division of the VIIIth cranial nerve, contains nerve fibers that originate from the neurons of the spiral ganglia located within small channels (*Rosenthal's canal*) at the root of each spiral lamina within the modiolus. They project peripherally to the cochlear hair cells in the cochlear duct and centrally through the small channels within the cribriform bone of the modiolus to the cochlear nuclei of the brainstem. A small posterior branch of the cochlear nerve supplies the vestibular end of the cochlear duct within the floor of the vestibule. The *vestibular nerve*, the other major trunk of the VIIIth cranial nerve, is composed of bipolar cells originating in the vestibular ganglion (*Scarpa's ganglion*) within the fundus of the IAC, sending efferent fibers to the neurosensory epithelium of the vestibular apparatus (utricle, saccule, and semicircular ampullae) and afferent fibers to the vestibular nuclei of the brainstem. It has an inferior and a superior division. The *inferior vestibular nerve* is composed of two branches, a posterior branch that innervates the ampullae of the posterior semicircular duct (Figs. 23, 24) and a saccular branch that innervates the saccular macula of the saccule. The *superior vestibular nerve* also has two branches, a utricular branch that innervates the macula of the utricle and an ampullary branch that supplies the ampullae of the superior and lateral semicircular ducts. The utricular branch enters the vestibule at the *vestibular pyramid,* which is a raised area of cribriform bone at the superior end of the *vestibular crest* (Fig. 21).

The cochlear nerve, inferior and superior divisions of the vestibular nerve, and facial nerve are arranged in separate quadrants within the IAC (Figs. 26–28). The canal is partitioned at its apex into superior and inferior halves by a horizontal bony shelf, the *crista falciformis* (Figs. 25–28), separating the facial nerve and superior division of the vestibular nerve superiorly from the cochlear nerve and inferior division of the vestibular nerve inferiorly. The superior half is further partitioned by *Bill's bar* (named after renowned

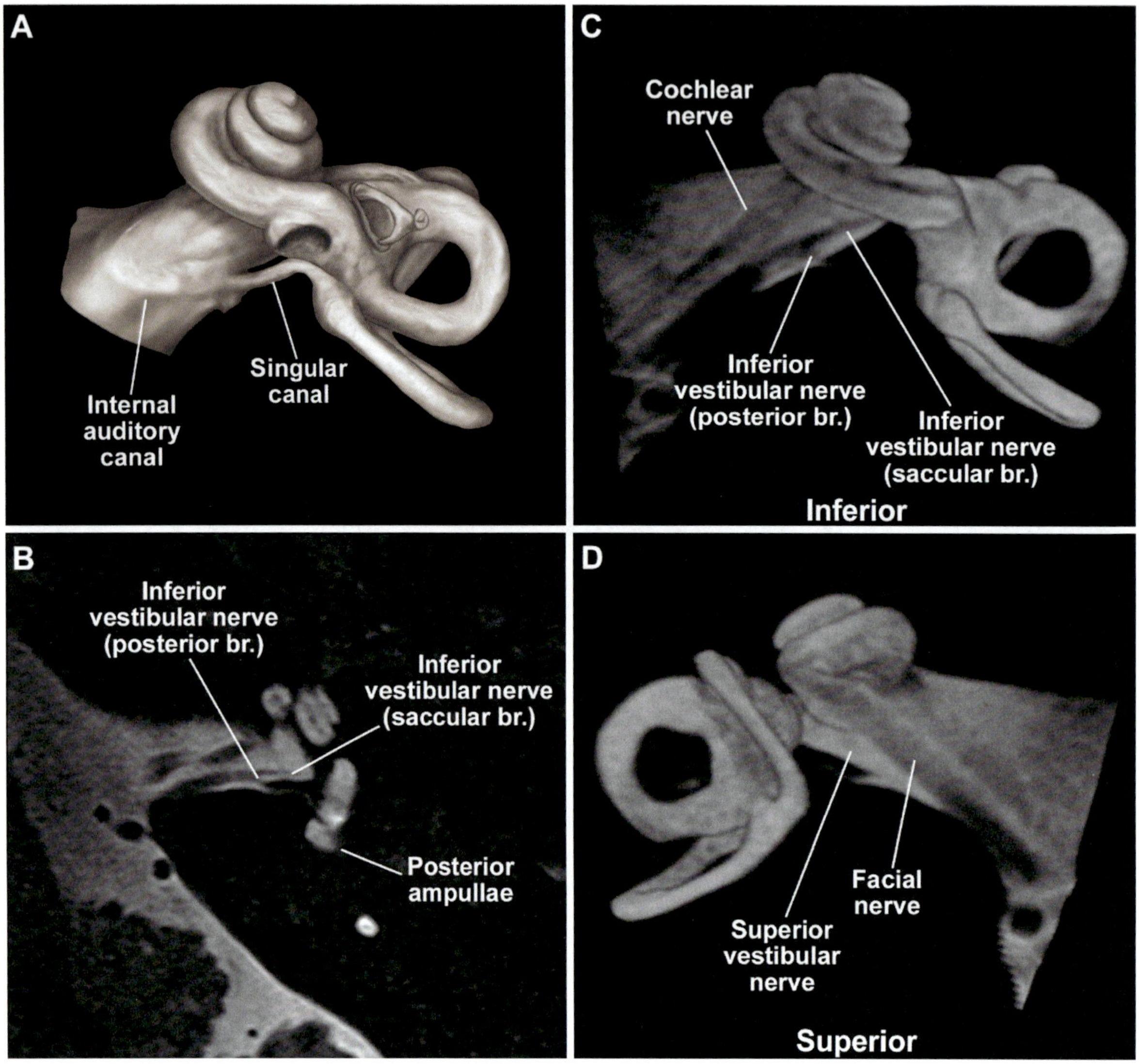

Fig. 24 IAC. (**a**) Inferior view of a 3D reconstruction from the microCT dataset demonstrating the relationship between the IAC and the bony labyrinth. Note the origin of the singular canal from the posterior wall of the IAC proximal to the apex. The singular canal transmits the posterior branch of the inferior vestibular nerve to the ampulla of the posterior semicircular duct. (**b**) 3T MR axial image demonstrates the length of the singular canal from its origin in the IAC to its entry at the base of the posterior ampulla. (**c**) Inferior view of 3D maximum intensity projection (MIP) reconstructed from 3T MR. Note the cochlear nerve anteriorly and both saccular and posterior branches of the inferior vestibular nerves posteriorly. (**d**) Superior view of 3D MIP reconstructed from 3T MR. Note the facial nerve anteriorly and the superior vestibular nerve posteriorly

neurotologist, Dr. William House), a vertically oriented crest of bone separating the facial nerve anteriorly from the superior vestibular nerve posteriorly (Fig. 27). The two branches of the inferior vestibular nerve transverse separate bony canals, the posterior branch transmitted to the posterior ampullae by way of the *singular canal* (Figs. 23, 24) and the saccular branch transmitted through a short foramen to the saccular macula (Fig. 23). The nerves exit the IAC through the *porus acusticus* on the posterior surface of the petrous portion of the temporal bone, superior and lateral to the opening of the *cochlear aqueduct* and superior and medial to the opening of the *vestibular aqueduct* (Fig. 28).

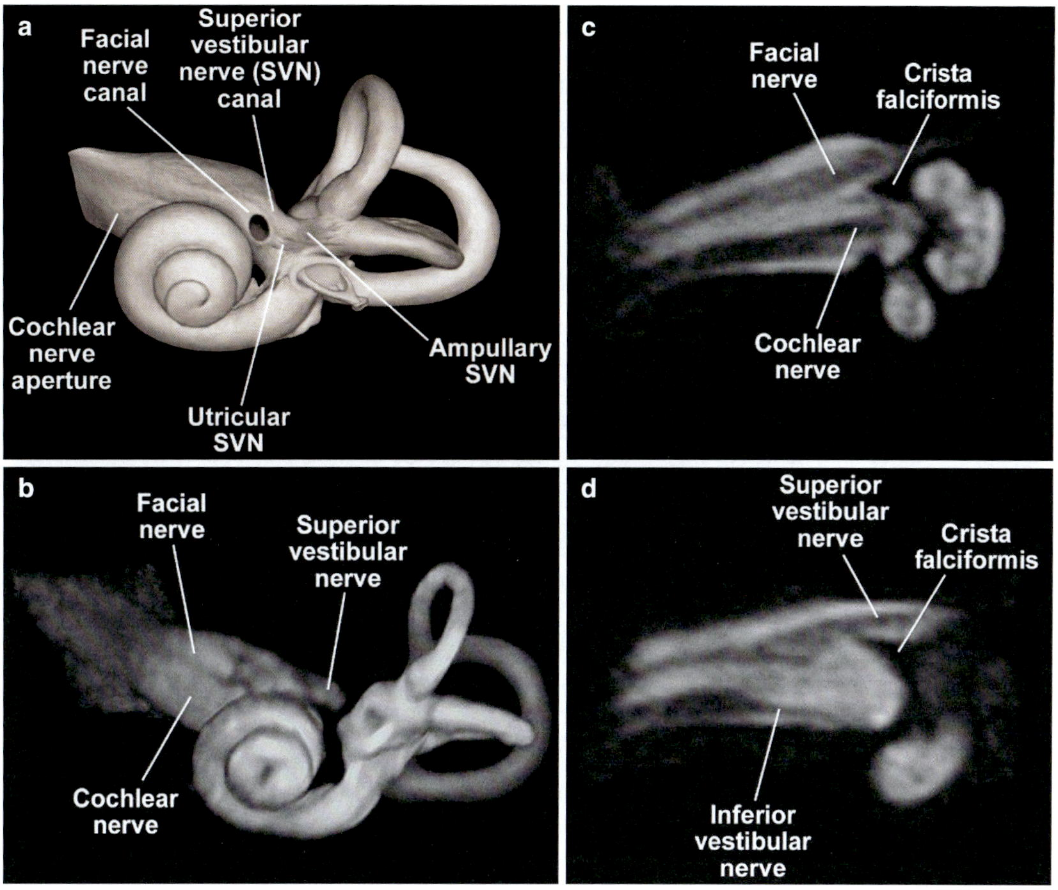

Fig. 25 IAC. (**a**) Anterior view of 3D reconstruction of the microCT dataset demonstrating the relationship between the IAC and the bony labyrinth. Note the cut surface of the labyrinthine segment of the facial nerve canal. The superior vestibular nerve canal can be seen to bifurcate into ampullary branches supplying the superior and lateral ampullae, and utricular branches inferiorly supplying the utricular macula. Note the cribriform bone at these sites of innervation. (**b**) 3D Maximum intensity projection (MIP) from in vivo 3T MR dataset in the same projection as (a). (**c**) Curved Multiplanar Reconstruction (MPR) of 3T MR along the course of the facial and cochlear nerves within the anterior IAC. (**d**) Curved MPR of 3T MR along the course of the vestibular nerves in the posterior IAC. Note the crista falciformis creating a bony partition at the IAC apex

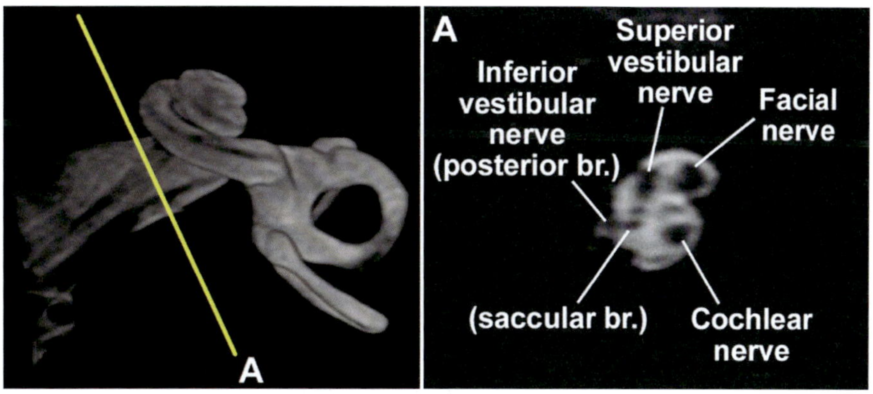

Fig. 26 IAC. Oblique cross-sectional reconstructions from in vivo 3T MR through the IAC demonstrating the relationship between the intracanalicular segments of the VIIth and VIIIth cranial nerves. (**a–e**) Progressive cross-sections from fundus to apex. Note the four-quadrant distribution of nerves within the fundus, with the facial nerve occupying the anterior–superior quadrant, the cochlear nerve in the anterior–inferior quadrant, the superior vestibular nerve in the posterior–superior quadrant, and the inferior vestibular nerve in the posterior–inferior quadrant (**a**). Also note the horizontal bony partition, the crista falciformis (**b**), and the superior vestibular nerve innervating the utricular macula (**e**)

Fig. 26 (continued)

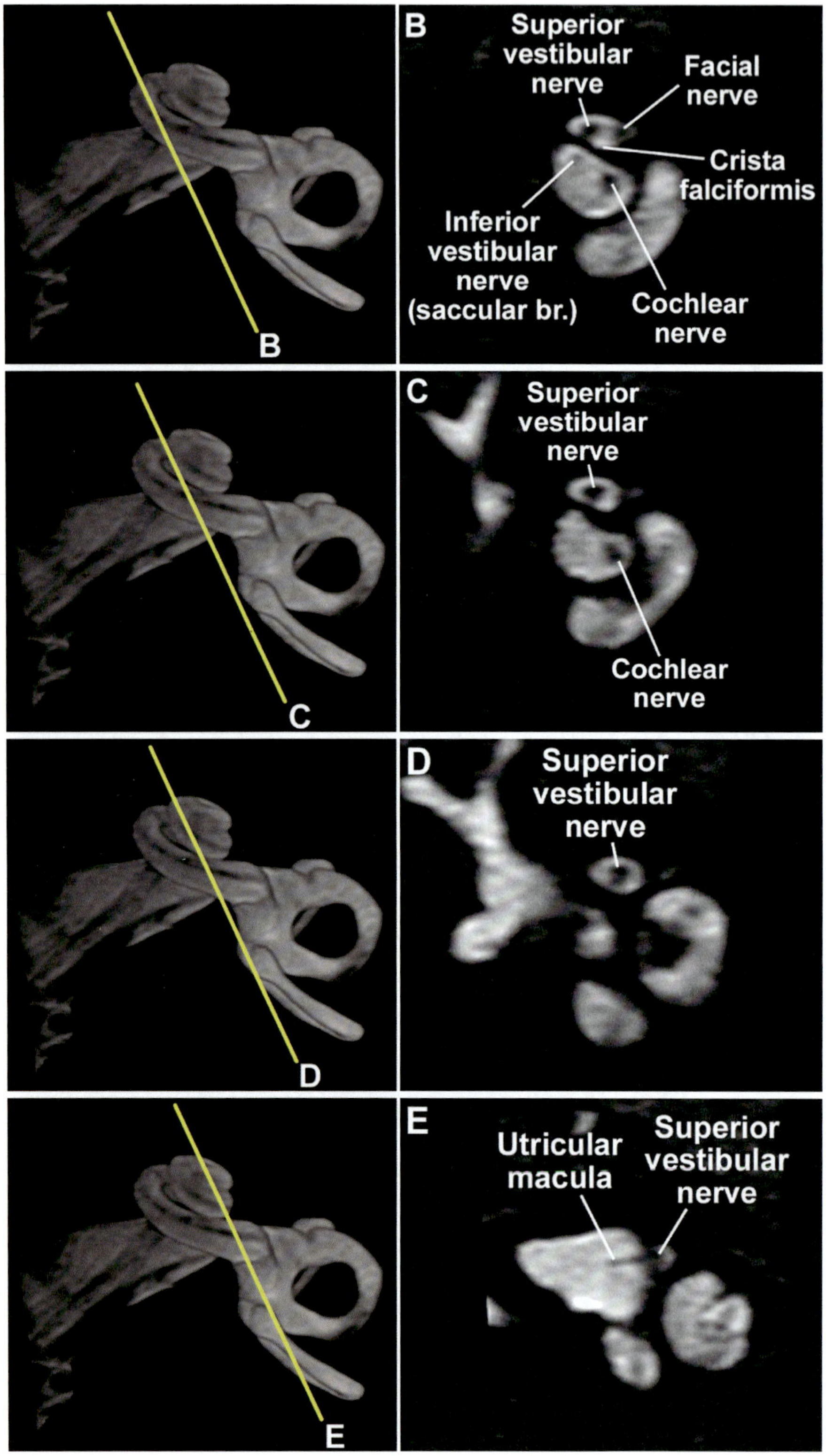

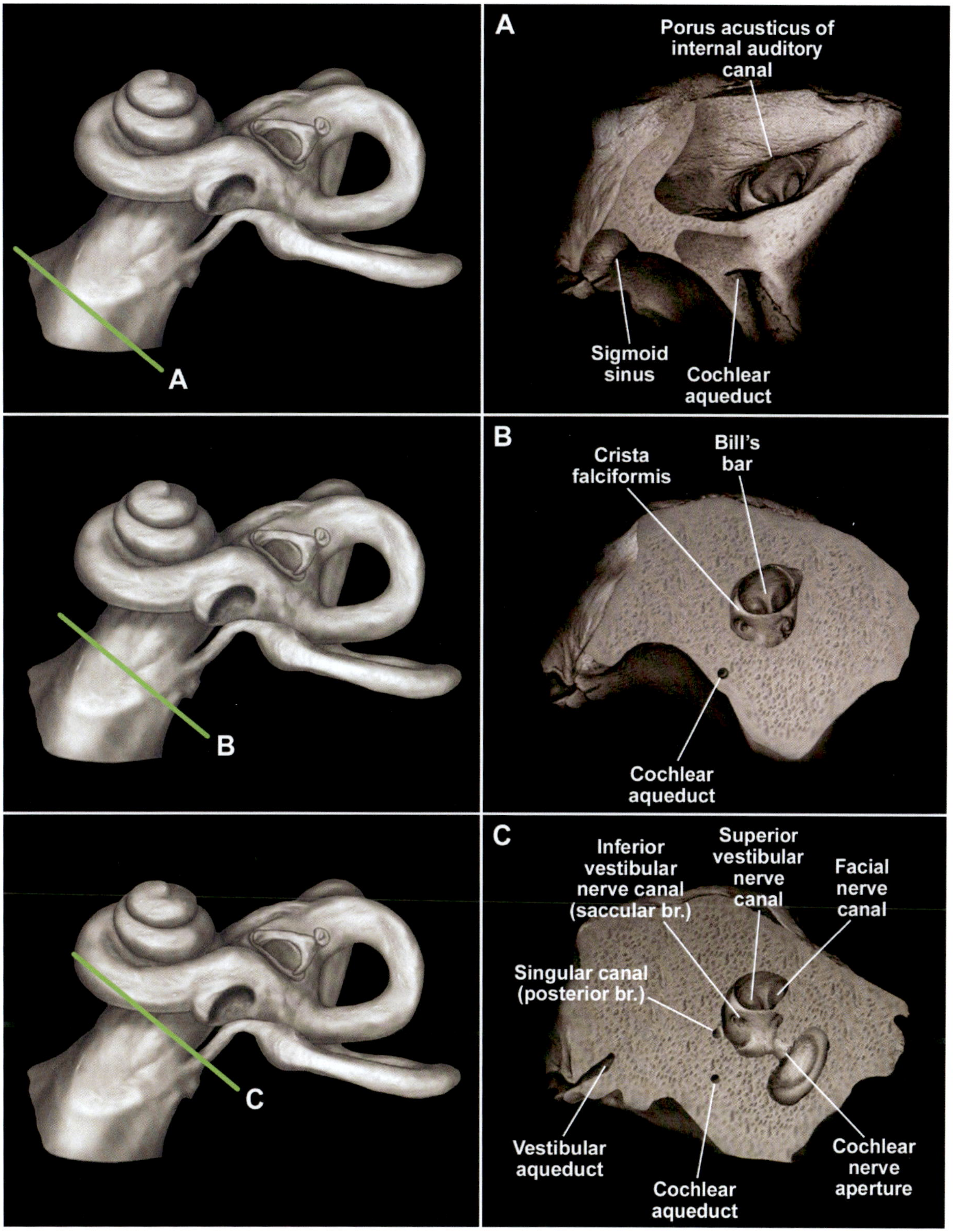

Fig. 27 IAC. Oblique cross-sectional reconstructions from the microCT dataset through the IAC demonstrating the exit points of the intracanalicular nerves into the bony labyrinth at the IAC apex. (**a–c**) Progressive cross-sections from the porus acusticus (the opening of the IAC) to the apex of the IAC. Note the horizontal and vertical divisions of the IAC by the crista falciformis and Bill's bar (after the renowned neurotologist Dr. William House) (**b**). Note the proximal exit of the posterior branch of the inferior vestibular nerve (supplying sensory fibers to the crista ampullaris of the posterior semicircular duct) by way of the singular canal (**c**)

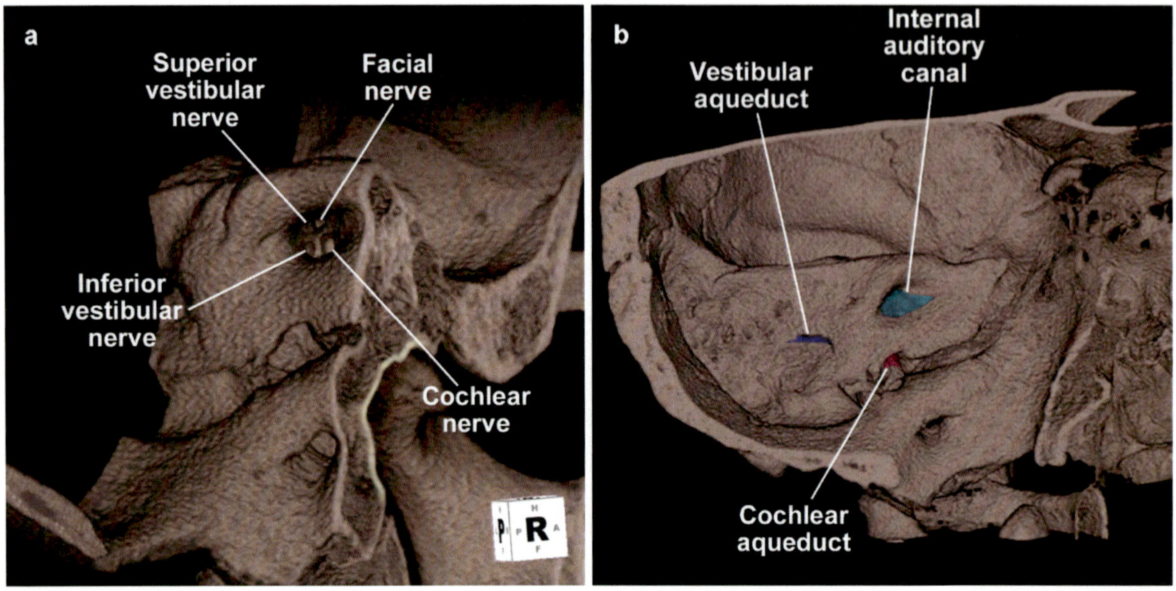

Fig. 28 IAC. Multidector CT reconstruction of the posteromedial surface of the petrous portion of the temporal bone. (**a**) Exposed view of the left IAC demonstrating nerve exit points at the IAC apex. (**b**) Posteromedial surface of the temporal bone demonstrating the location of the porus acusticus of the IAC in relation to the opening of the cochlear aqueduct inferiorly and the opening of the vestibular aqueduct posteriorly

Reference

1. Gopen Q, Rosowski JJ, Merchant SN. Anatomy of the normal human cochlear aqueduct with functional implications. *Hear Res* 1997;107:9–22

Multiplanar Atlas

3

In this chapter, images of the temporal bone will be displayed in four planes of section using four imaging modalities. Cadaver specimens were used to acquire volumetric acquisitions with microCT and microMR. Sixty-four slice multidetector CT (MDCT) and 3T MR were used to acquire the in vivo images (techniques previously discussed in Chap. 1). All imaging planes were reconstructed from the original volumetric acquisitions into the axial (in the plane of the lateral semicircular canal), coronal (perpendicular to the lateral semicircular canal), Pöschl (short axis temporal bone), and Stenvers (long axis temporal bone) planes with the exception of the 3T imaging in which images were acquired in all four planes of presentation. Although the four images were matched as closely as possible, this was not always exact because of normal anatomical variations (both the cadaver and in vivo images were acquired using different subjects).

Temporal Bone Imaging: Historical Perspectives

Temporal bone imaging became a specialized area of study in radiology with the advent of polytomography during the late 1950s and early 1960s. The recommended tube angulation for these examinations was dependent on the anatomical region of greatest clinical interest with frontal (coronal) and lateral (sagittal) projections comprising the standard examination [1]. Supplementary projections were developed to show certain structures to better advantage. The Stenvers projection, a long axis view of the petrous portion of the temporal bone, was used to profile, among other structures, the round window and posterior semicircular canal. The Pöschl projection, a short axis view of the petrous pyramid, was used to optimally visualize the superior semicircular canal, anterior wall of the cochlea and vestibular aqueduct [2, 3]. With the advent of computerized tomography, the restrictions imposed by limitations in gantry angle defined the axial and coronal planes as the standard views, replacing the older standard tomographic planes. With single slice CT or 2D MR, the plane of section was determined manually at the console before the scan was acquired. The development of isotropic volumetric acquisitions with both CT as well as MR has obviated the need for detailed attention to the plane of acquisition since the plane of section can be determined in the post-processing phase of the examination. The imager can ensure the reproducibility of the standard planes of section by defining these planes with reference to fixed anatomical structures. In our practice, we have defined the axial plane as being parallel to that of the lateral semicircular canal, with the coronal plane being oriented exactly perpendicular to the axial plane. Additionally, the Pöschl and Stenvers planes can be reconstructed along the short and long axes of the petrous portion of the temporal bone and used as an adjunct to the axial and coronal planes.

J. I. Lane, R. J. Witte, *The Temporal Bone*, DOI: 10.1007/978-3-642-02210-4_3,

The Axial Plane (in the Plane of the Lateral Semicircular Canal)

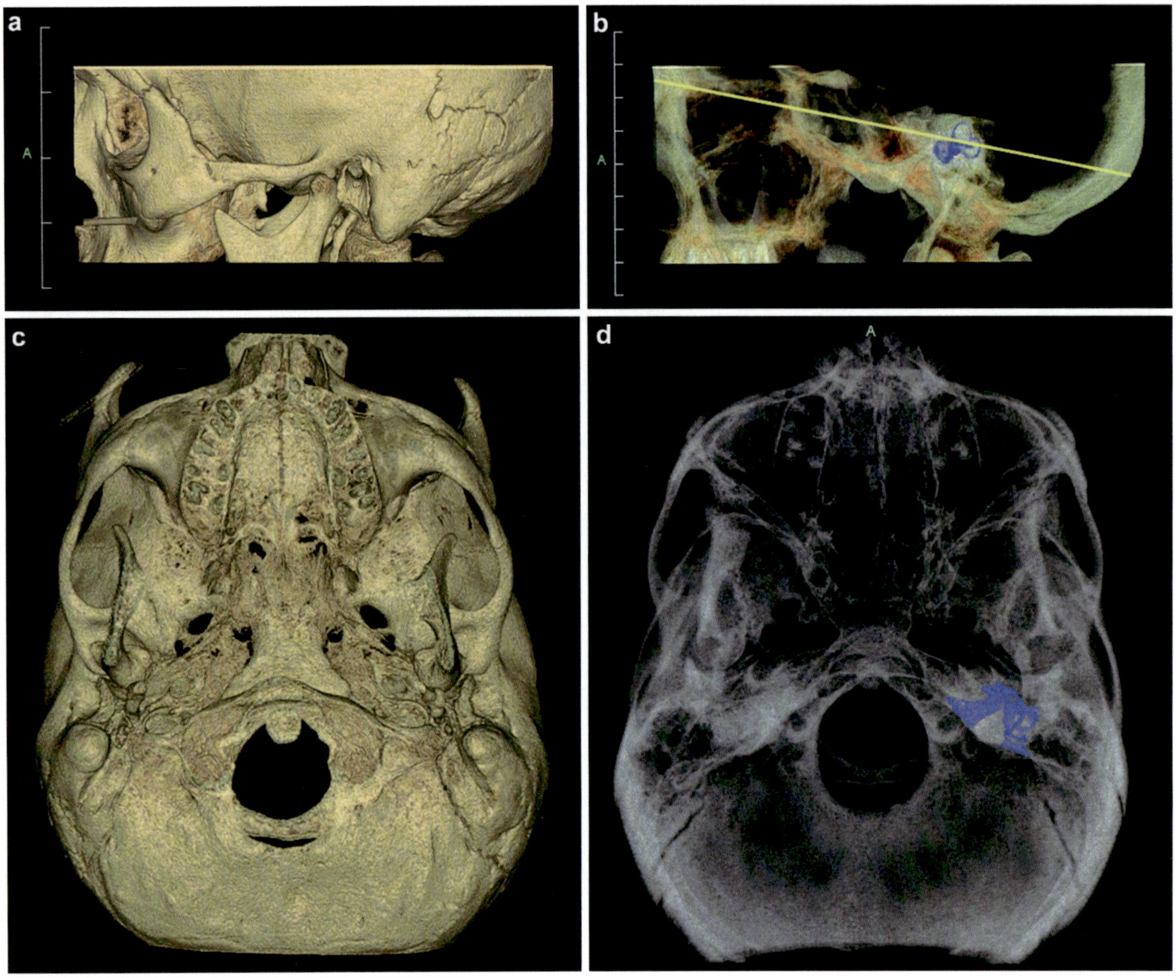

Fig. 1 Axial plane of section through the left temporal bone. (**a**) Lateral view of 3D surface-rendered reconstruction from multidetector CT (MDCT) volume. (**b**) Maximum intensity projection with color-segmented labyrinth showing orientation of lateral semicircular canal. *Yellow line* indicates plane of section parallel to lateral semicircular canal. (**c**) Inferior view of 3D surface-rendered reconstruction from MDCT volume oriented in the axial plane of section. (**d**) Maximum intensity projection demonstrating orientation of the labyrinth in the axial plane

The following serial images in the axial plane are presented from inferior to superior to include microCT (*upper left*), MDCT (*upper right*), microMR (*lower left*), and 3T MR (*lower right*).

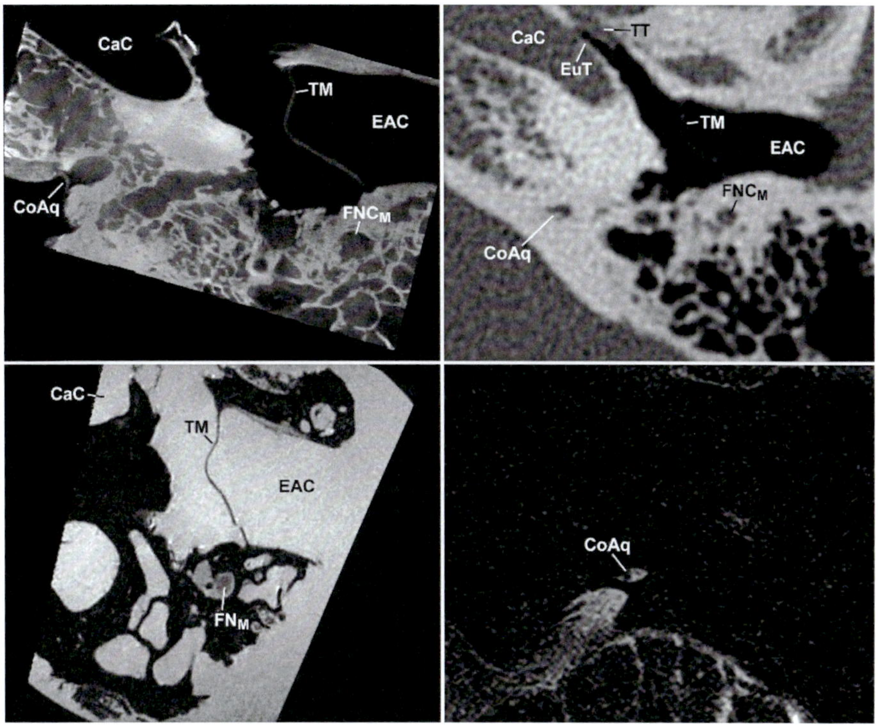

Fig. 2

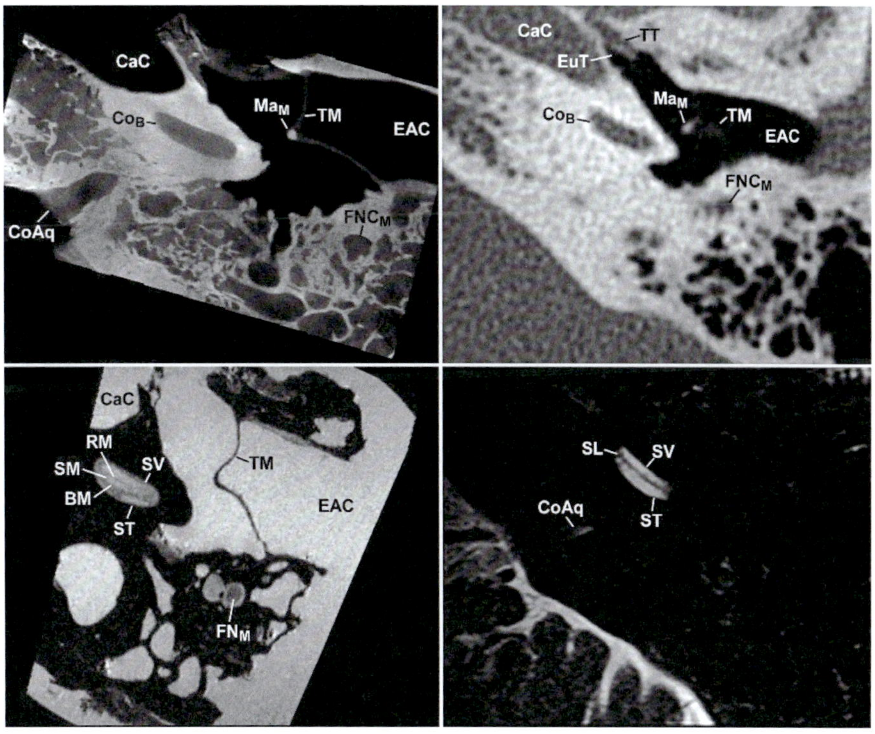

Fig. 3

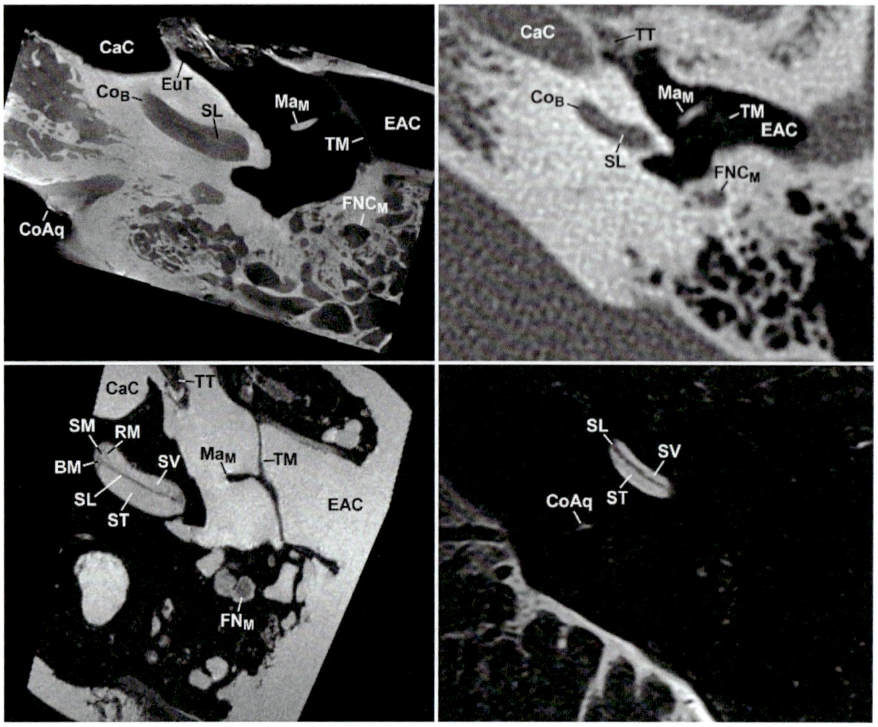
CaC
EuT
CoB
SL
MaM
EAC
TM
FNCM
CoAq
TT
CaC
CoB
MaM
TM
EAC
SL
FNCM
CaC
TT
SM
RM
BM
SV
MaM
TM
SL
ST
EAC
FNM
SL
SV
CoAq
ST

Fig. 4

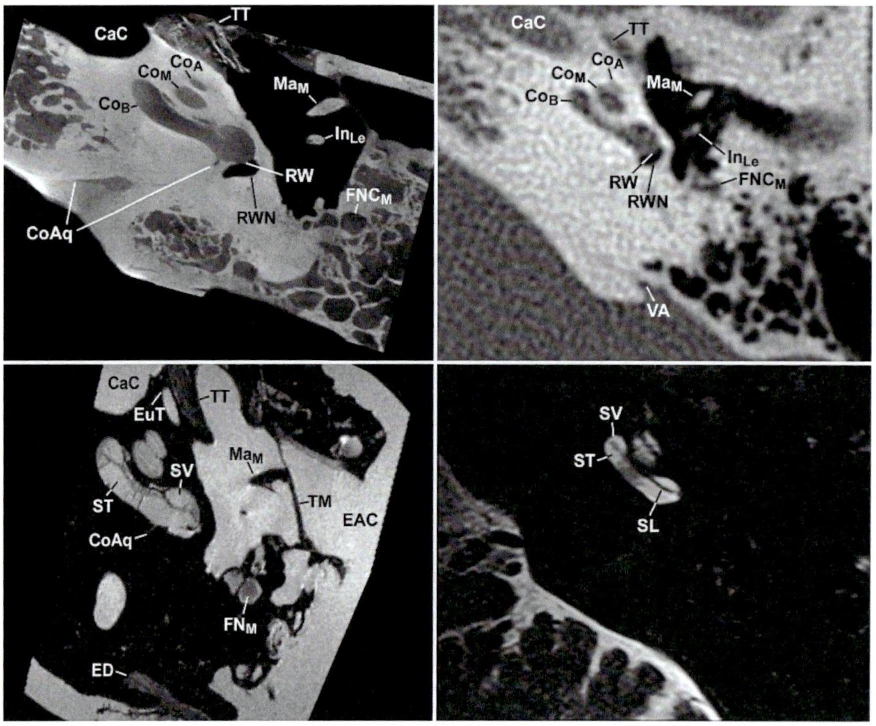
TT
CaC
CoA
CoM
MaM
CoB
InLe
RW
RWN
FNCM
CoAq
CaC
TT
CoA
CoM
CoB
MaM
InLe
RW
RWN
FNCM
VA
CaC
EuT
TT
MaM
SV
ST
TM
EAC
CoAq
FNM
ED
SV
ST
SL

Fig. 5

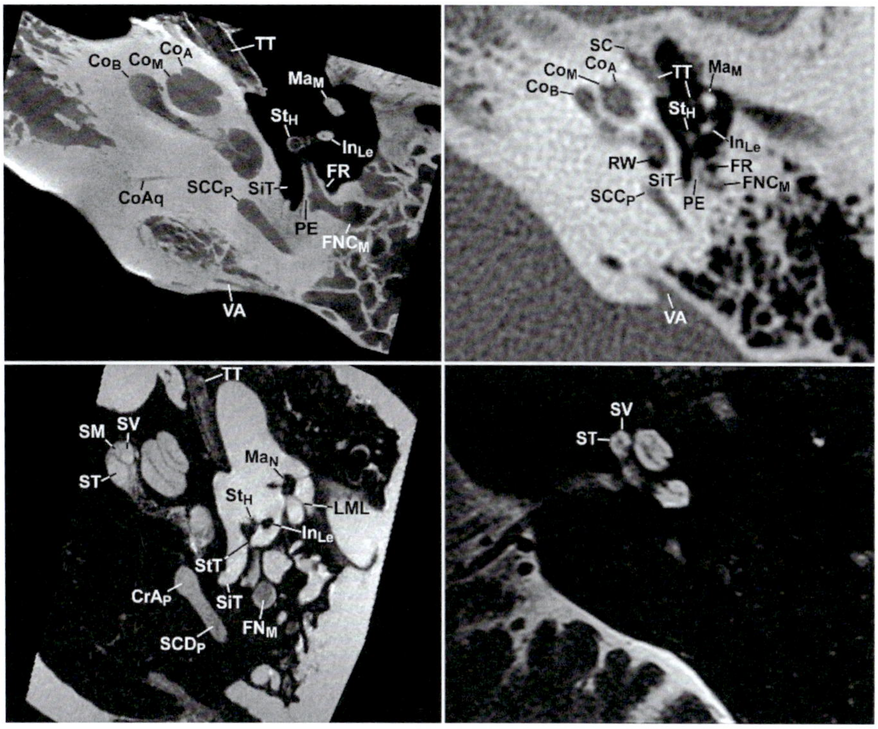
TT
CoA
CoB
CoM
MaM
StH
InLe
FR
CoAq
SCCP
SiT
PE
FNCM
VA
SC
RW
SM
SV
ST
MaN
LML
StT
CrAP
FNM
SCDP
Fig. 6

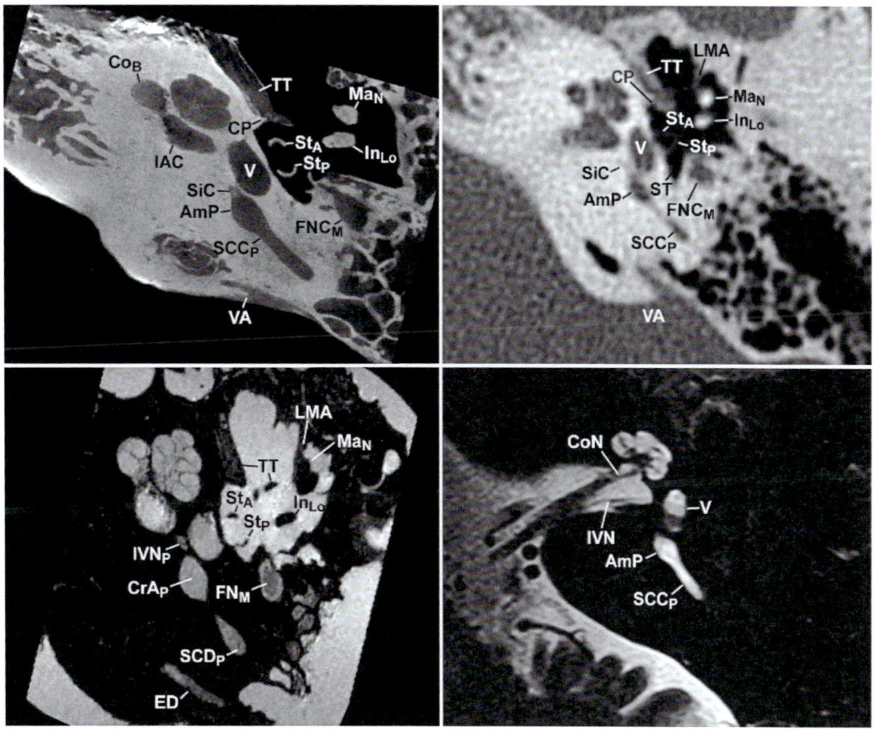
CoB
TT
MaN
CP
StA
InLo
StP
IAC
V
SiC
AmP
FNCM
SCCP
VA
LMA
ST
IVNP
CrAP
FNM
SCDP
ED
CoN
IVN
Fig. 7

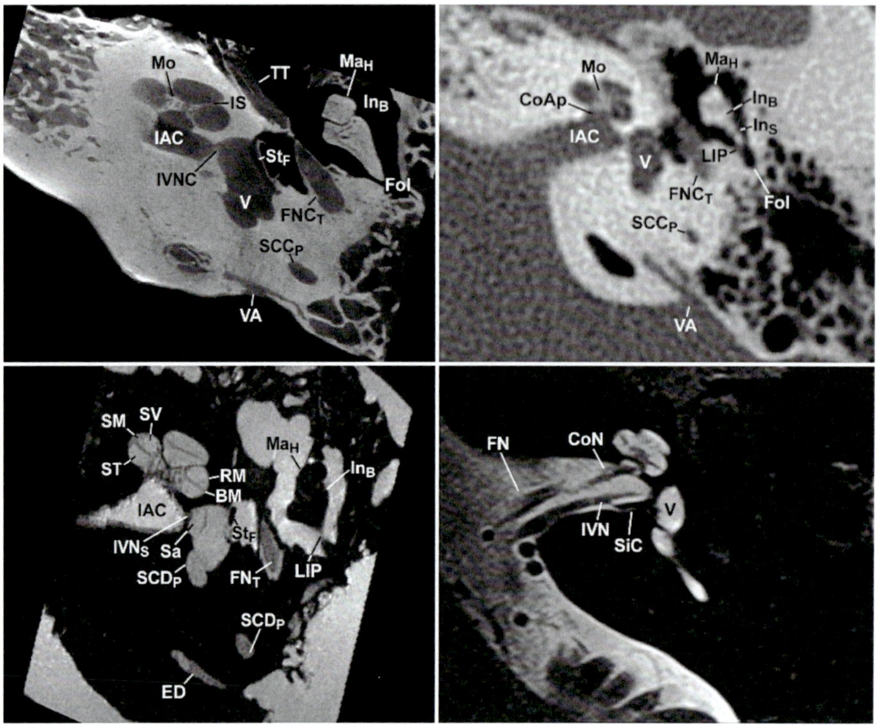
Mo
TT
MaH
IS
InB
IAC
StF
IVNC
Fol
V
FNCT
SCCP
VA
Mo
MaH
CoAp
InB
InS
IAC
V
LIP
FNCT
Fol
SCCP
VA
SM
SV
MaH
ST
RM
InB
BM
IAC
StF
IVNS
Sa
SCDP
FNT
LIP
SCDP
ED
FN
CoN
V
IVN
SiC

Fig. 8

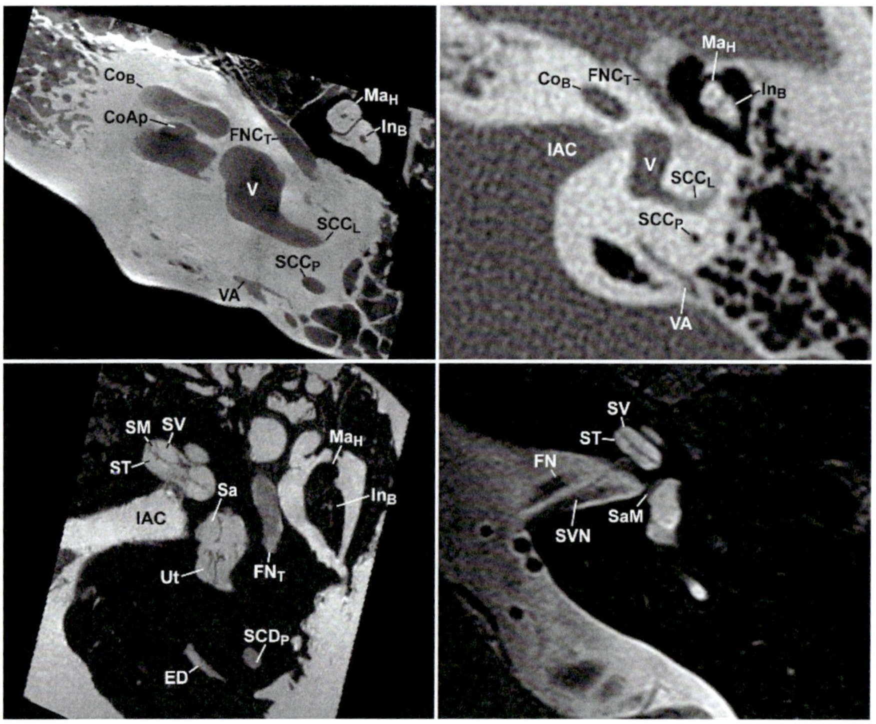
CoB
MaH
CoAp
InB
FNCT
V
SCCL
SCCP
VA
MaH
CoB
FNCT
InB
IAC
V
SCCL
SCCP
VA
SM
SV
MaH
ST
Sa
InB
IAC
Ut
FNT
SCDP
ED
SV
ST
FN
SaM
SVN

Fig. 9

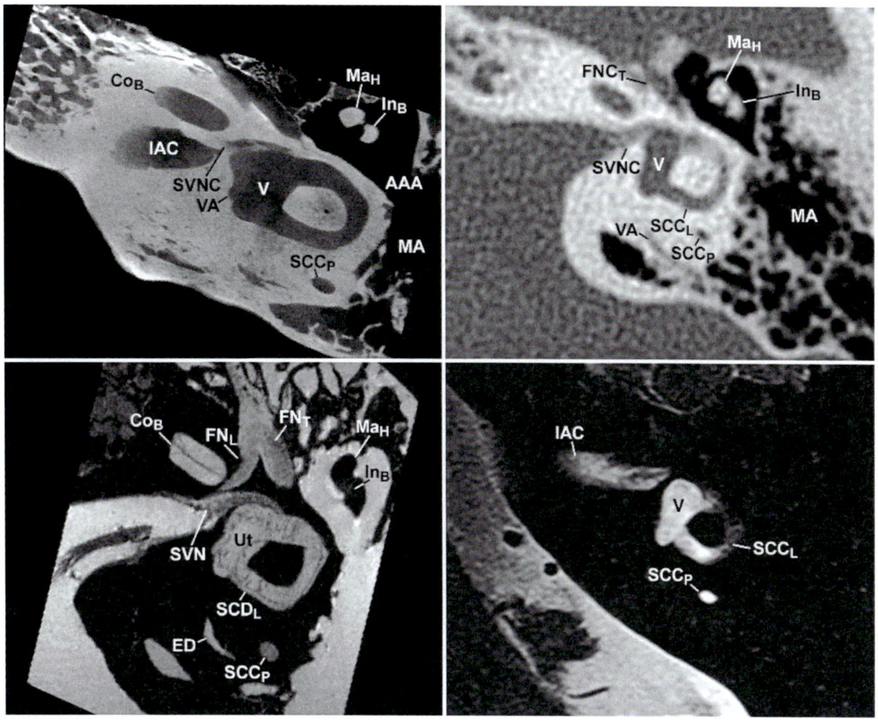
CoB
MaH
InB
IAC
SVNC
V
VA
AAA
MA
SCCP
FNCT
SCCL
FNL
FNT
Ut
SVN
SCDL
ED

Fig. 10

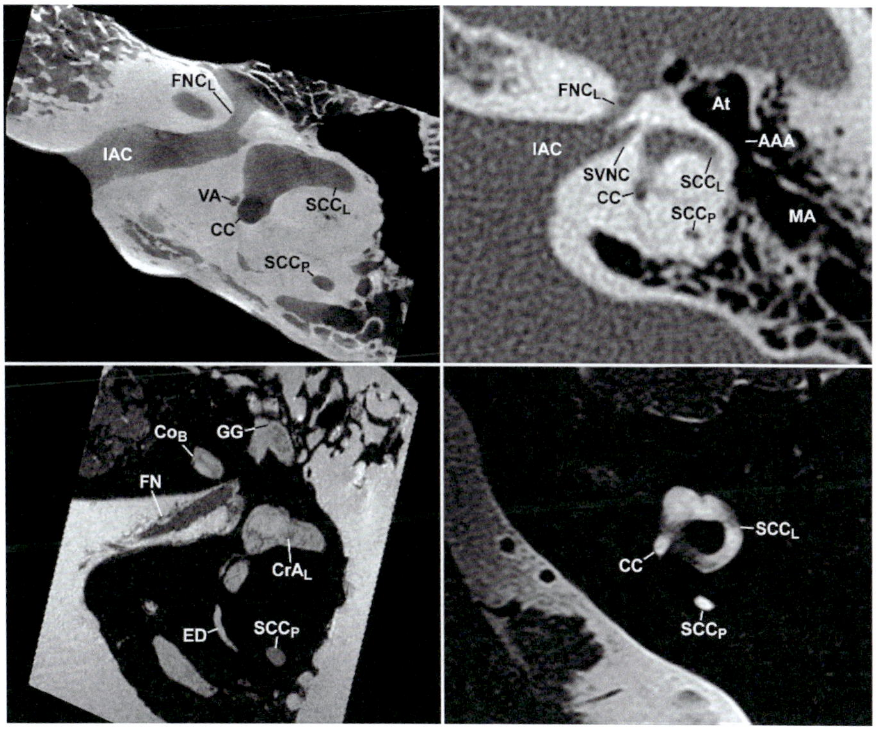
FNCL
IAC
VA
CC
SCCL
SCCP
At
AAA
SVNC
MA
CoB
GG
FN
CrAL
ED

Fig. 11

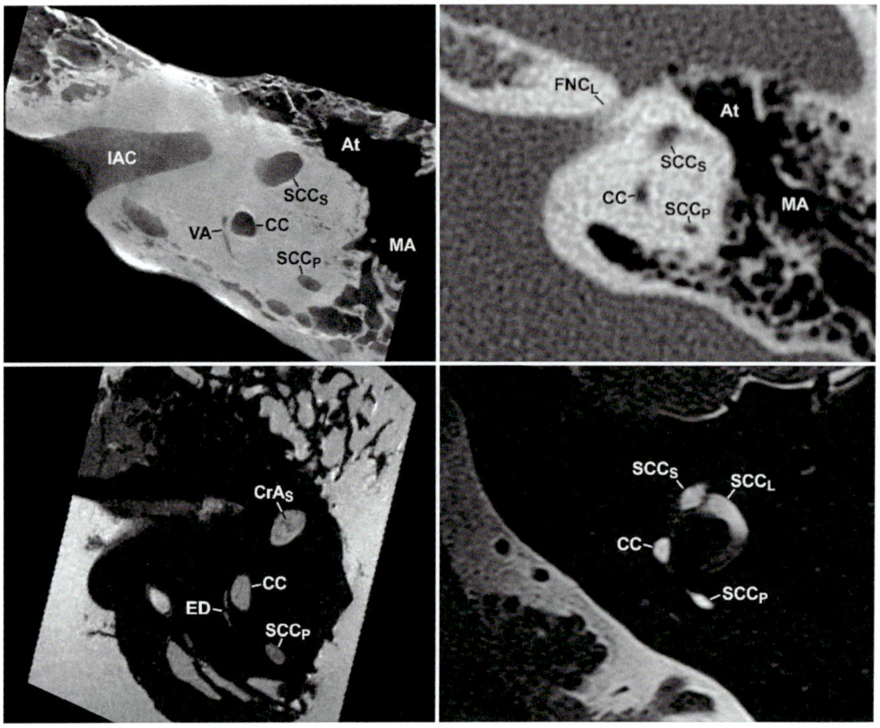
IAC
At
SCCs
VA
CC
SCCP
MA
FNCL
At
SCCs
CC
SCCP
MA
CrAs
CC
ED
SCCP
SCCs
SCCL
CC
SCCP

Fig. 12

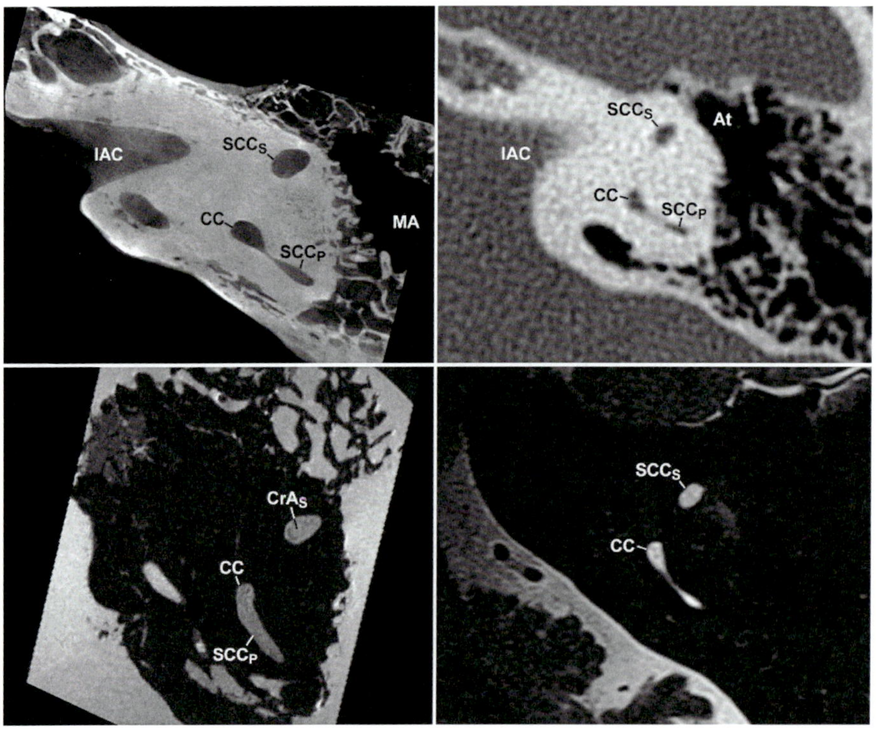
IAC
SCCs
CC
SCCP
MA
SCCs
At
IAC
CC
SCCP
CrAs
CC
SCCP
SCCs
CC

Fig. 13

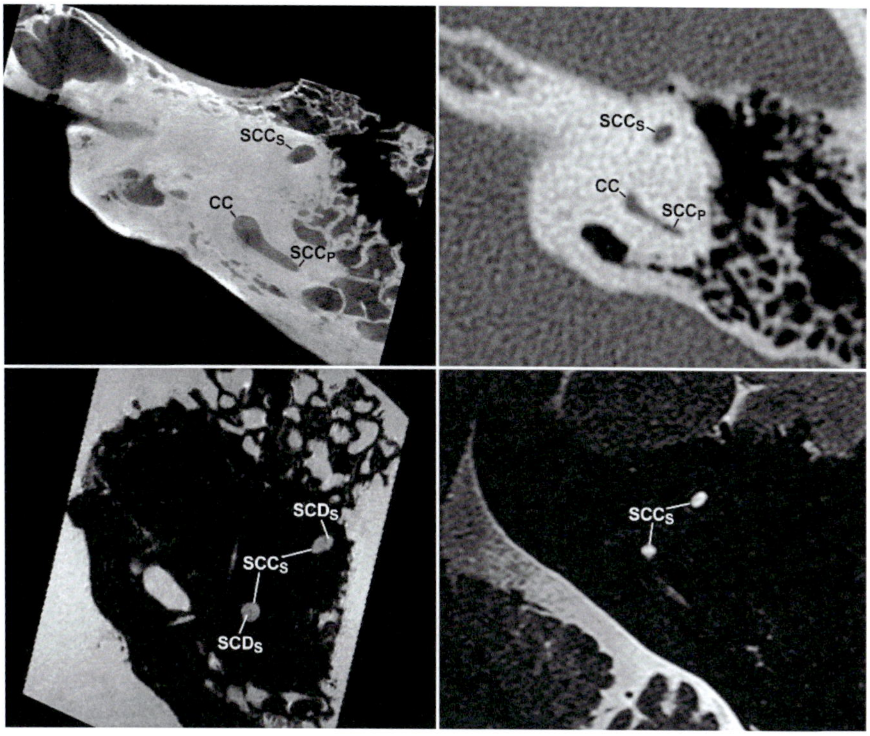
SCCs
CC
SCCp
SCCs
CC
SCCp
SCDs
SCCs
SCDs
SCCs

Fig. 14

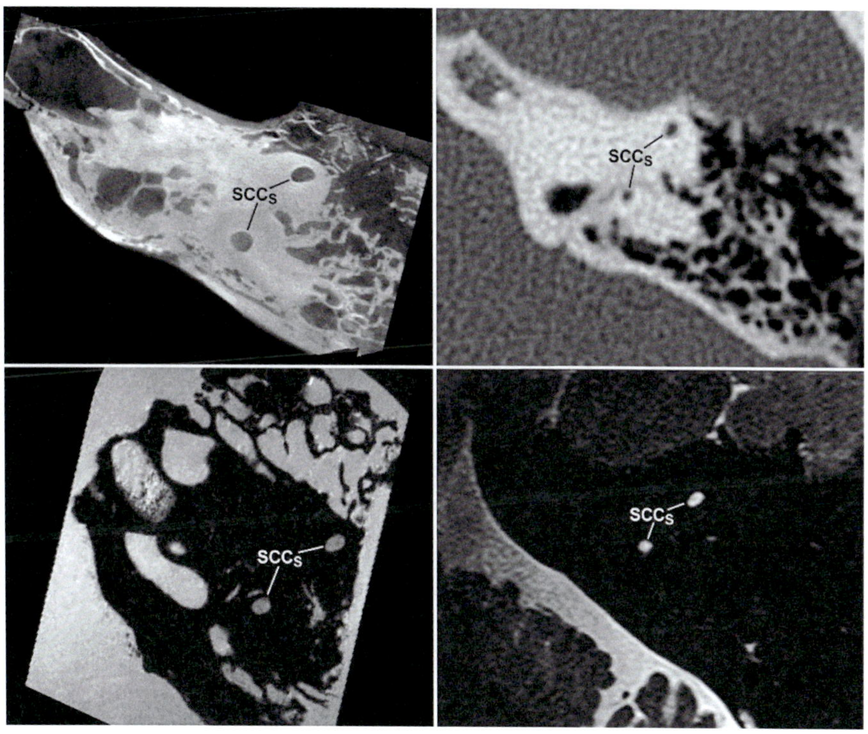
SCCs
SCCs
SCCs
SCCs

Fig. 15

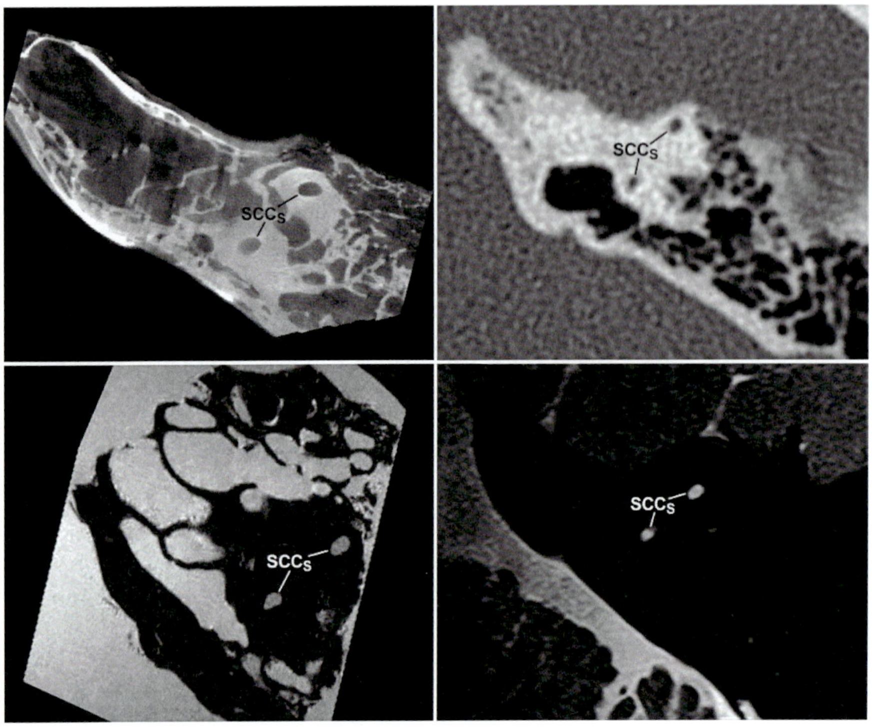

Fig. 16

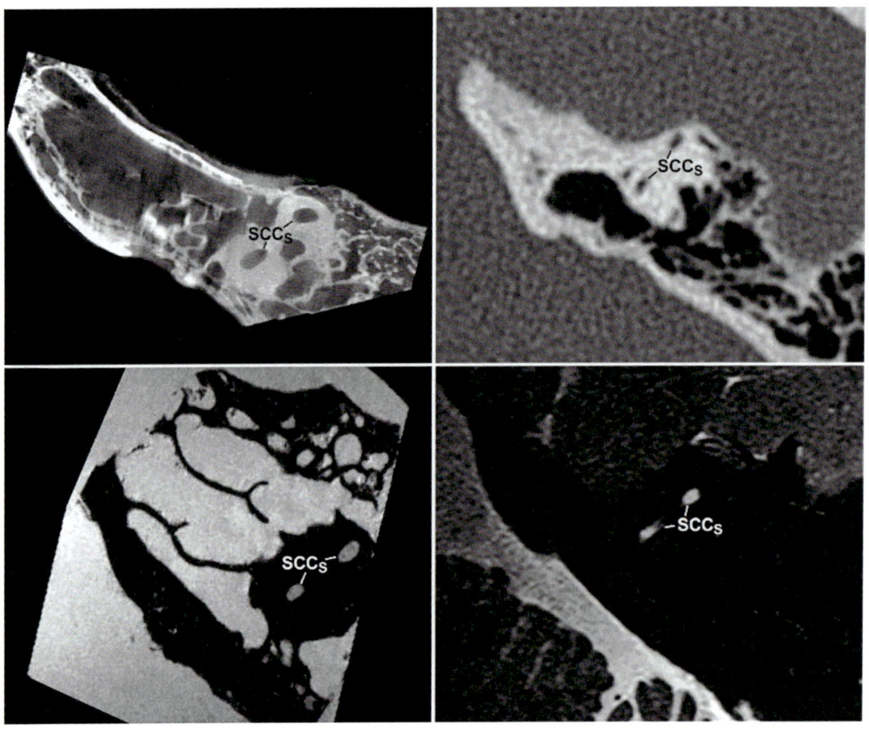

Fig. 17

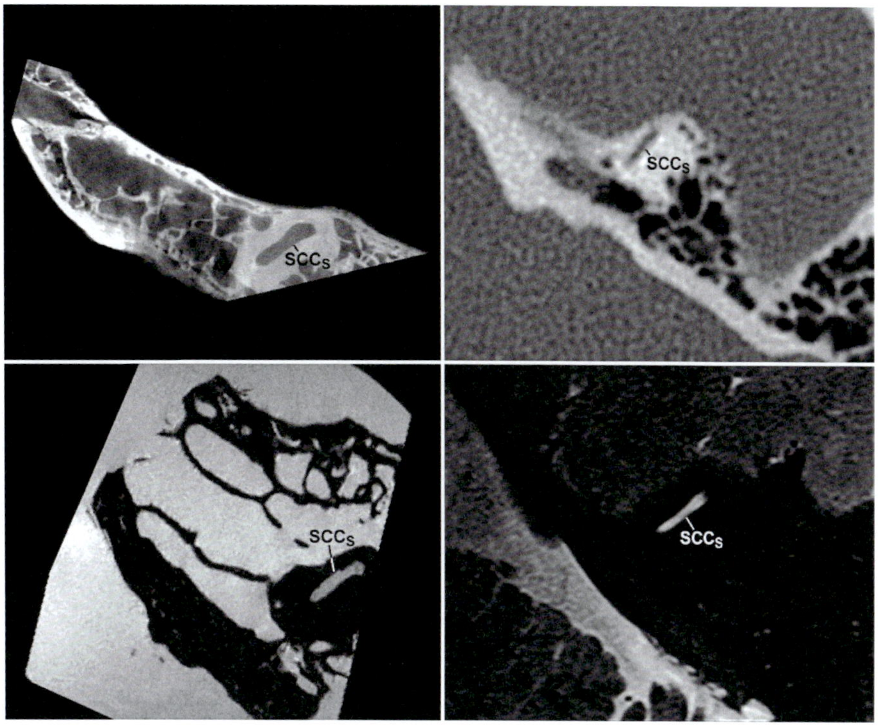

Fig. 18

The Coronal Plane (Perpendicular to the Plane of the Lateral Semicircular Canal)

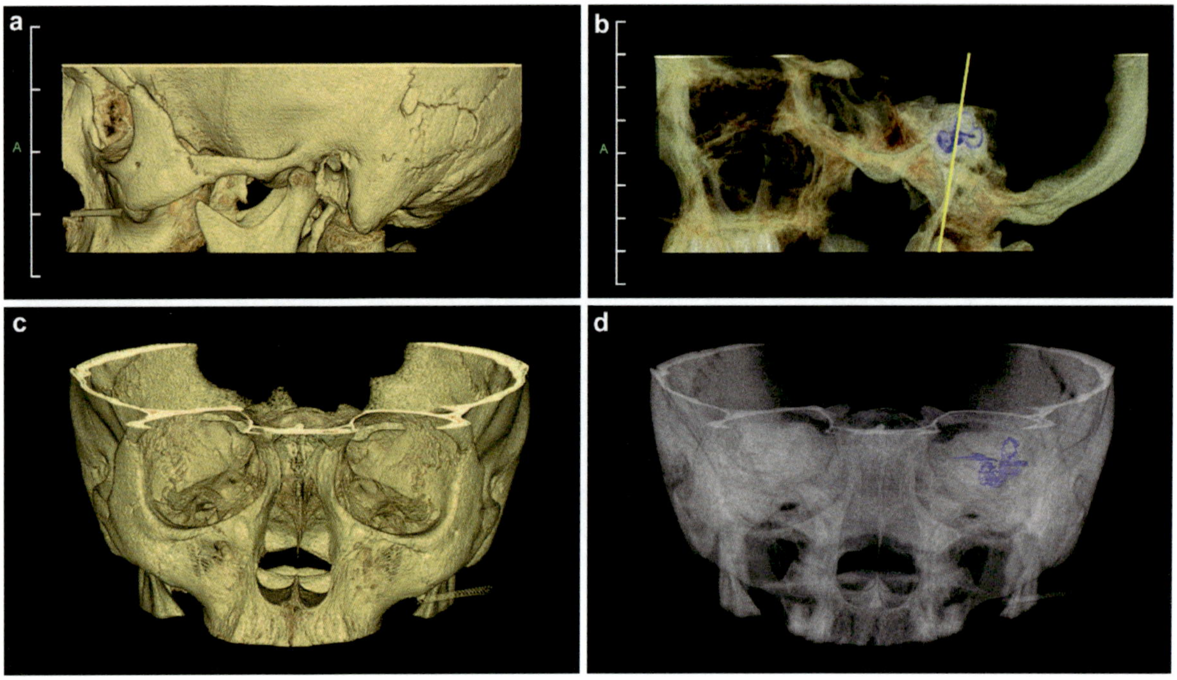

Fig. 19 Coronal plane of section through the left temporal bone. (**a**) Lateral view of 3D surface-rendered reconstruction from MDCT volume. (**b**) Maximum intensity projection with color-segmented labyrinth showing orientation of the lateral semicircular canal. *Yellow line* indicates the plane of section perpendicular to the lateral semicircular canal. (**c**) Anterior view of 3D surface-rendered reconstruction from MDCT volume oriented in the coronal plane of section. (**d**) Maximum intensity projection demonstrating orientation of the labyrinth in the coronal plane

The following serial images in the coronal plane are presented from anterior to posterior to include microCT (*upper left*), MDCT (*upper right*), microMR (*lower left*), and 3T MR (*lower right*).

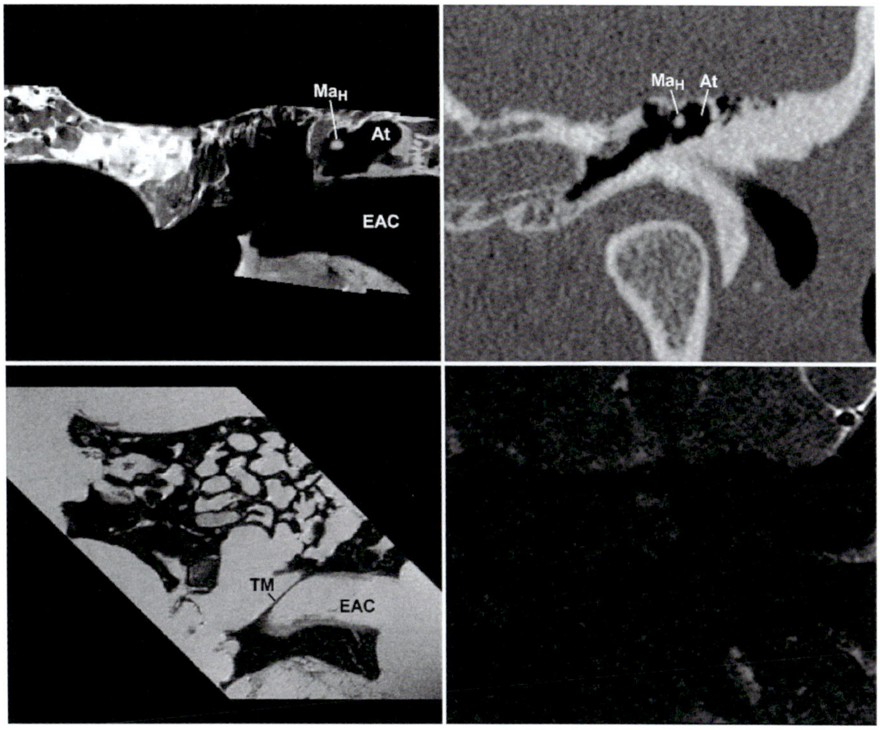

Fig. 20

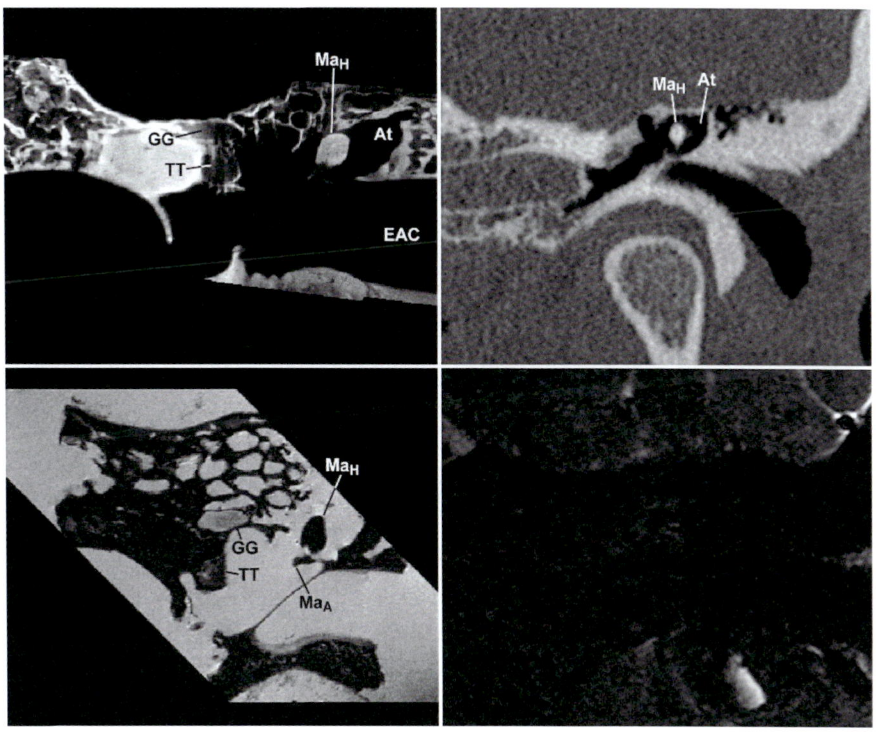

Fig. 21

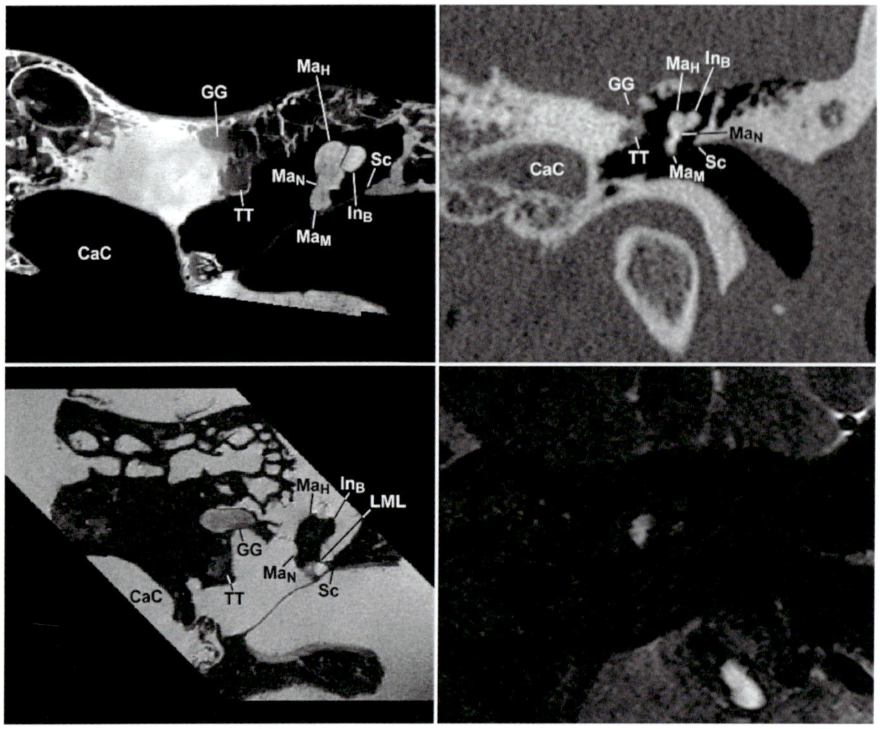
MaH
GG
Sc
MaN
TT
InB
MaM
CaC
MaH
InB
GG
MaN
TT
Sc
CaC
MaM
MaH
InB
LML
GG
MaN
CaC
TT
Sc

Fig. 22

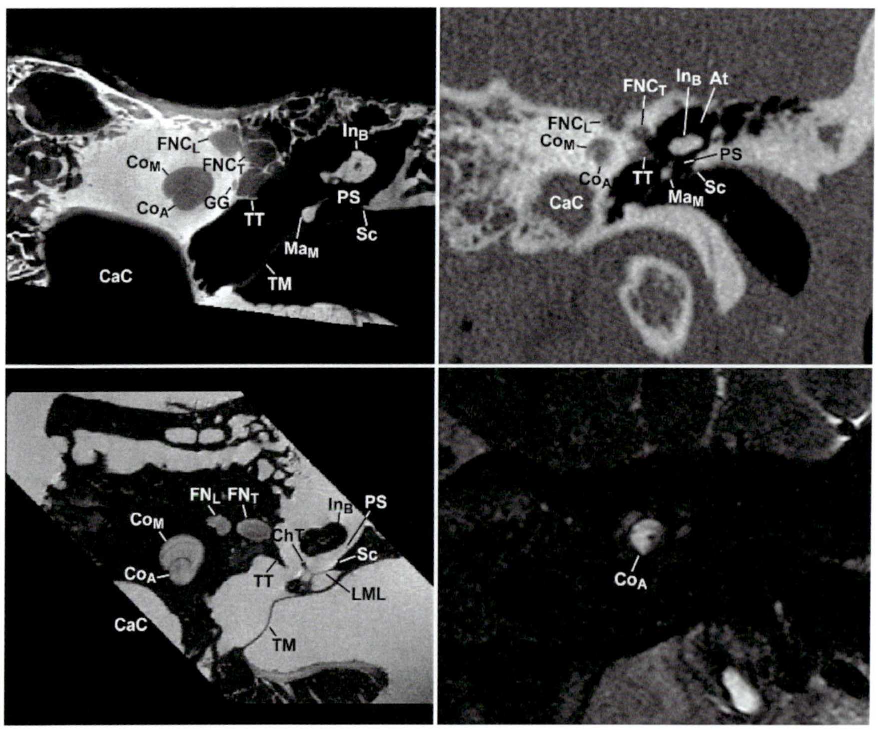
InB
FNCL
CoM
FNCT
CoA
GG
TT
PS
Sc
MaM
CaC
TM
FNCT
InB
At
FNCL
CoM
PS
CoA
TT
Sc
MaM
CaC
FNL
FNT
InB
PS
CoM
ChT
Sc
CoA
TT
LML
CaC
TM
CoA

Fig. 23

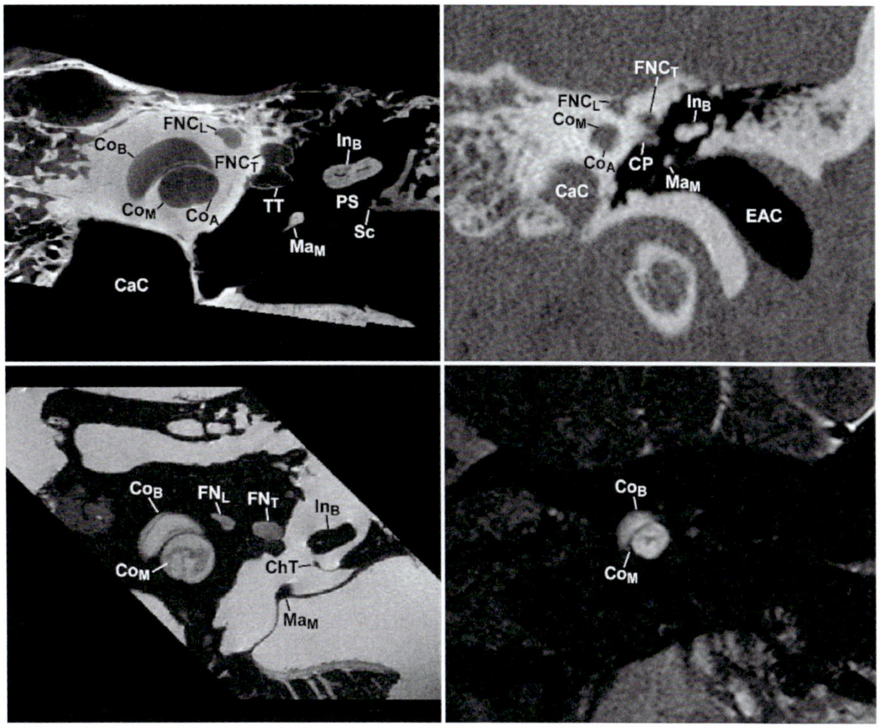
FNCL
CoB
FNCT
InB
CoM
CoA
TT
PS
Sc
MaM
CaC
FNCT
FNCL
CoM
InB
CoA
CP
MaM
CaC
EAC
CoB
FNL
FNT
InB
CoM
ChT
MaM
CoB
CoM

Fig. 24

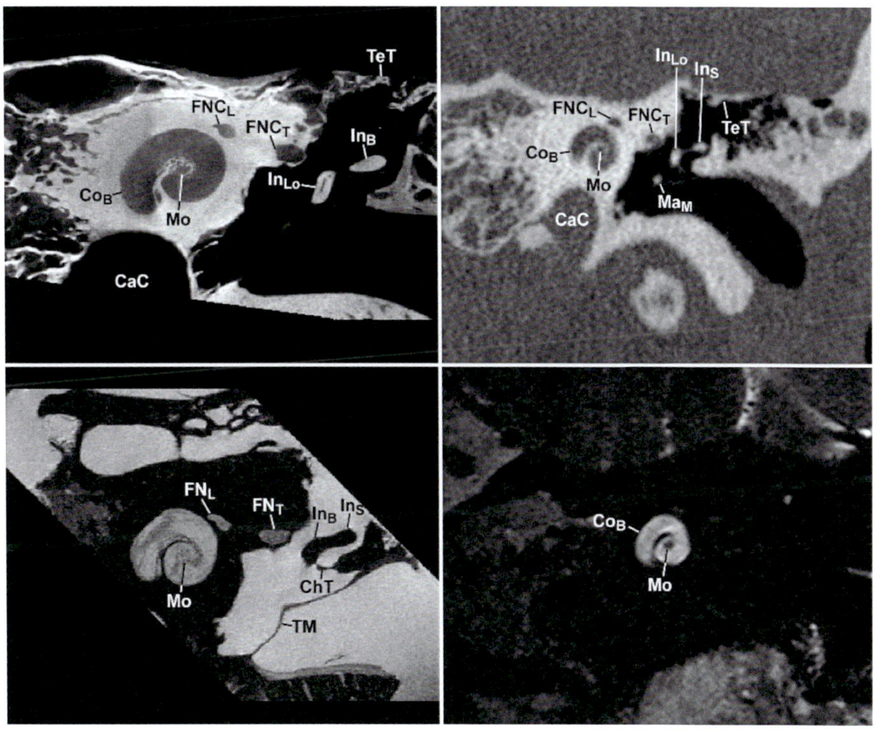
TeT
FNCL
FNCT
InB
InLo
CoB
Mo
CaC
InLo
InS
FNCL
FNCT
TeT
CoB
Mo
MaM
CaC
FNL
FNT
InB
InS
Mo
ChT
TM
CoB
Mo

Fig. 25

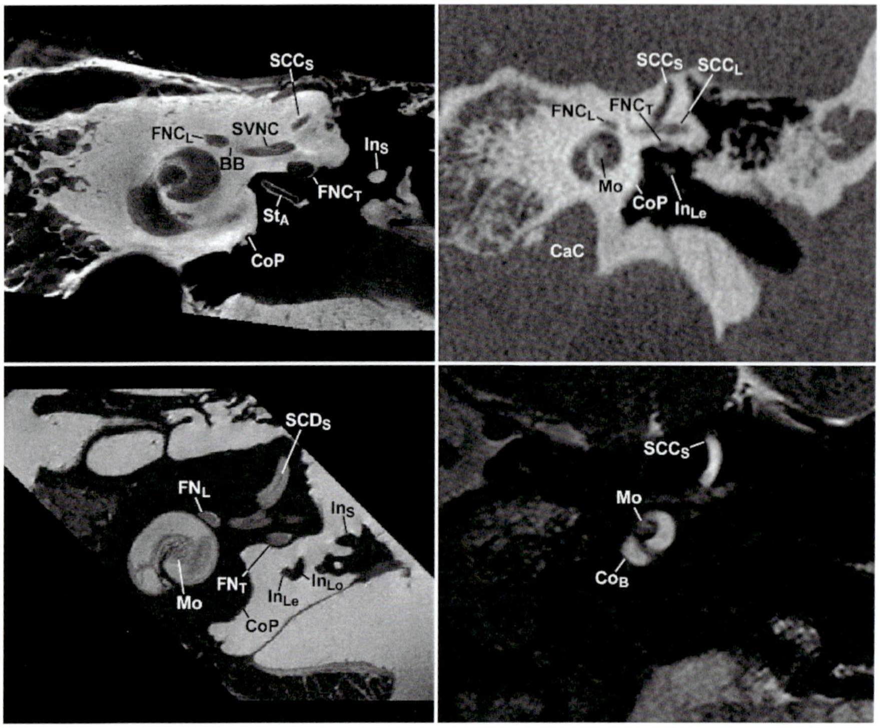
SCCS
FNCL
SVNC
BB
InS
FNCT
StA
CoP
SCCS
SCCL
FNCL
FNCT
Mo
CoP
InLe
CaC
SCDS
FNL
InS
InLo
FNT
InLe
Mo
CoP
SCCS
Mo
CoB

Fig. 26

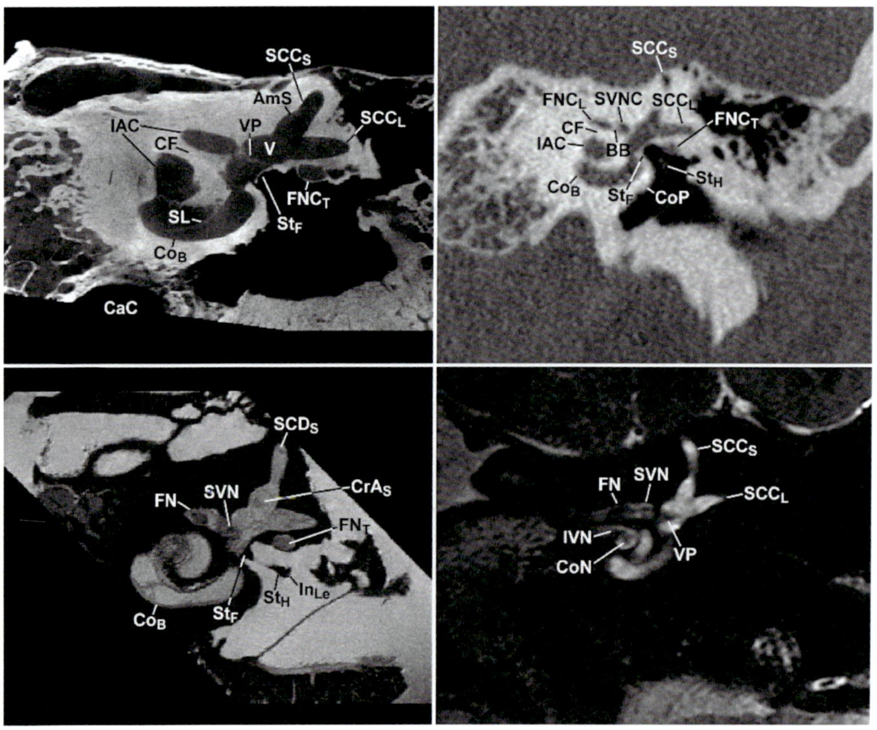
SCCS
AmS
IAC
VP
SCCL
CF
V
FNCT
StF
SL
CoB
CaC
SCCS
FNCL
SVNC
SCCL
FNCT
CF
IAC
BB
StH
CoB
StF
CoP
SCDS
CrAS
FN
SVN
FNT
StH
InLe
CoB
StF
SCCS
FN
SVN
SCCL
IVN
VP
CoN

Fig. 27

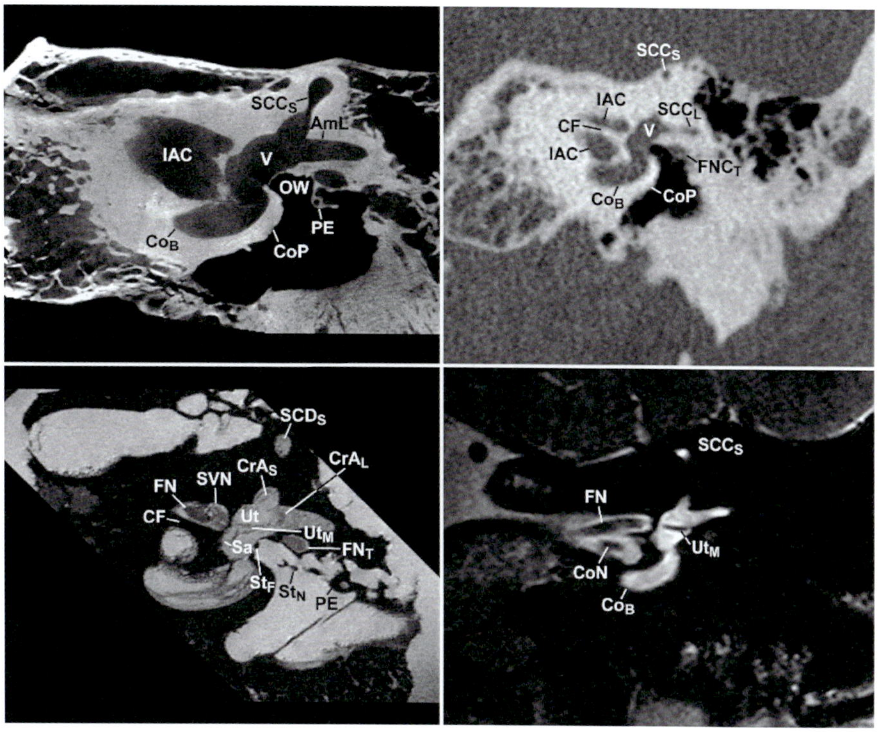
SCC_S
AmL
IAC
V
OW
PE
Co_B
CoP
SCC_S
IAC
SCC_L
CF
V
IAC
FNC_T
Co_B
CoP
SCD_S
CrA_L
CrA_S
FN
SVN
CF
Ut
Ut_M
Sa
FN_T
St_F
St_N
PE
SCC_S
FN
Ut_M
CoN
Co_B

Fig. 28

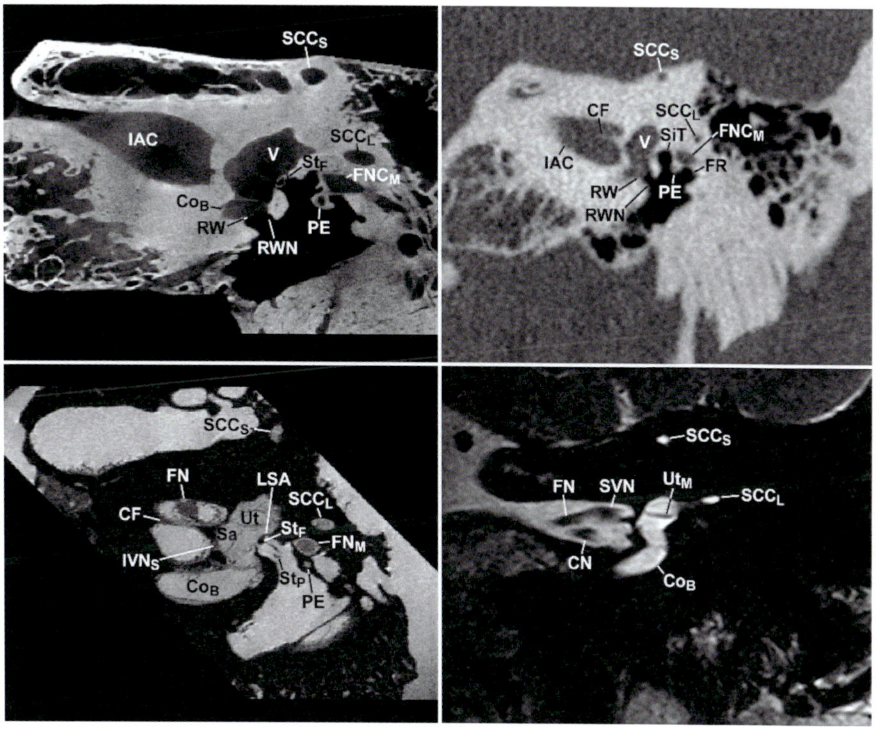
SCC_S
IAC
SCC_L
V
St_F
FNC_M
Co_B
RW
PE
RWN
SCC_S
CF
SCC_L
V
SiT
FNC_M
IAC
FR
RW
PE
RWN
SCC_S
FN
LSA
SCC_L
CF
Ut
Sa
St_F
FN_M
IVN_S
St_P
Co_B
PE
SCC_S
FN
SVN
Ut_M
SCC_L
CN
Co_B

Fig. 29

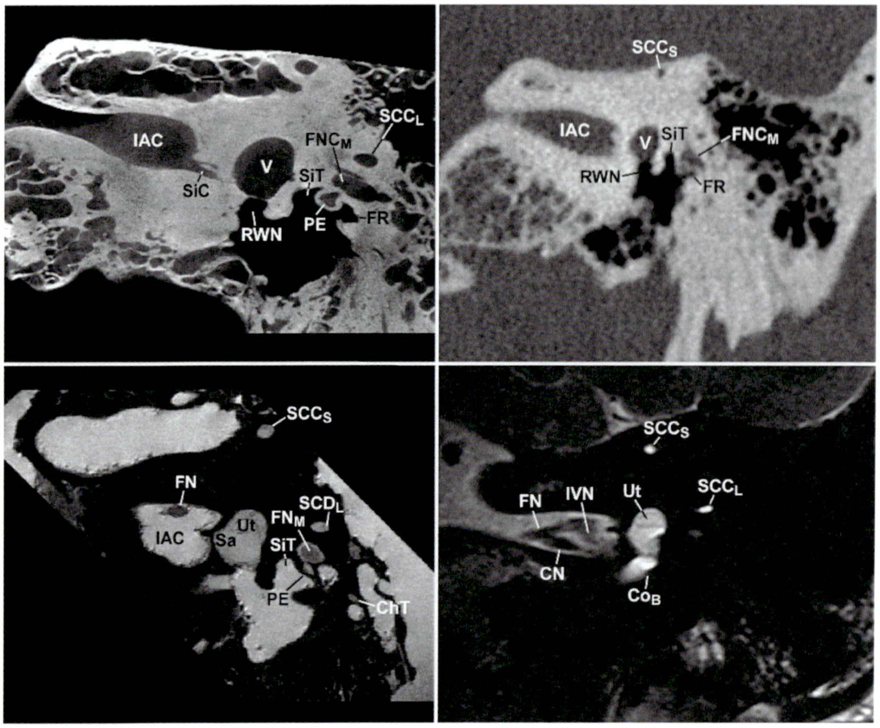
SCCL
IAC
FNCM
V
SiT
SiC
RWN
PE
FR
SCCS
IAC
SiT
FNCM
V
RWN
FR
SCCS
FN
SCDL
Ut
FNM
IAC
Sa
SiT
PE
ChT
SCCS
FN
IVN
Ut
SCCL
CN
CoB

Fig. 30

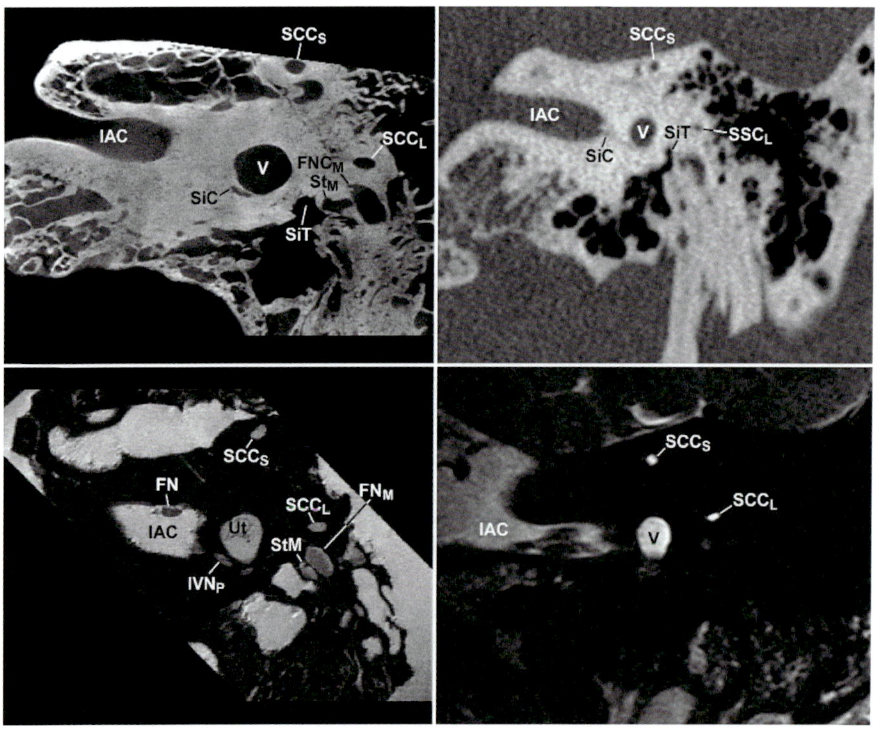
SCCS
IAC
SCCL
V
FNCM
StM
SiC
SiT
SCCS
IAC
V
SiT
SSCL
SiC
SCCS
FN
FNM
SCCL
IAC
Ut
StM
IVNP
SCCS
SCCL
IAC
V

Fig. 31

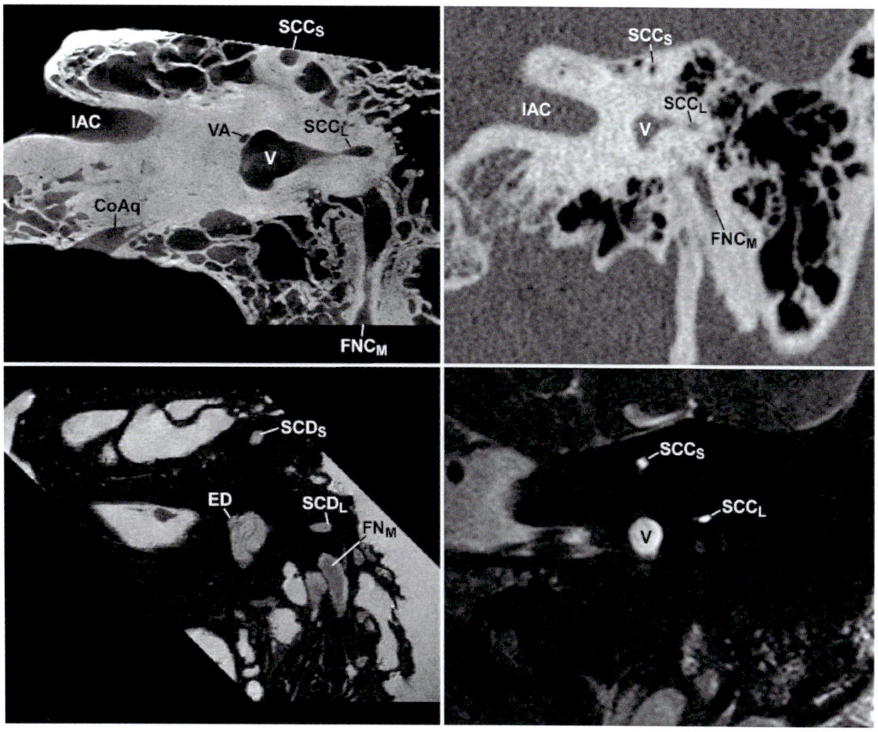
SCC$_S$
IAC
VA
V
SCC$_L$
CoAq
FNC$_M$
SCD$_S$
ED
SCD$_L$
FN$_M$

Fig. 32

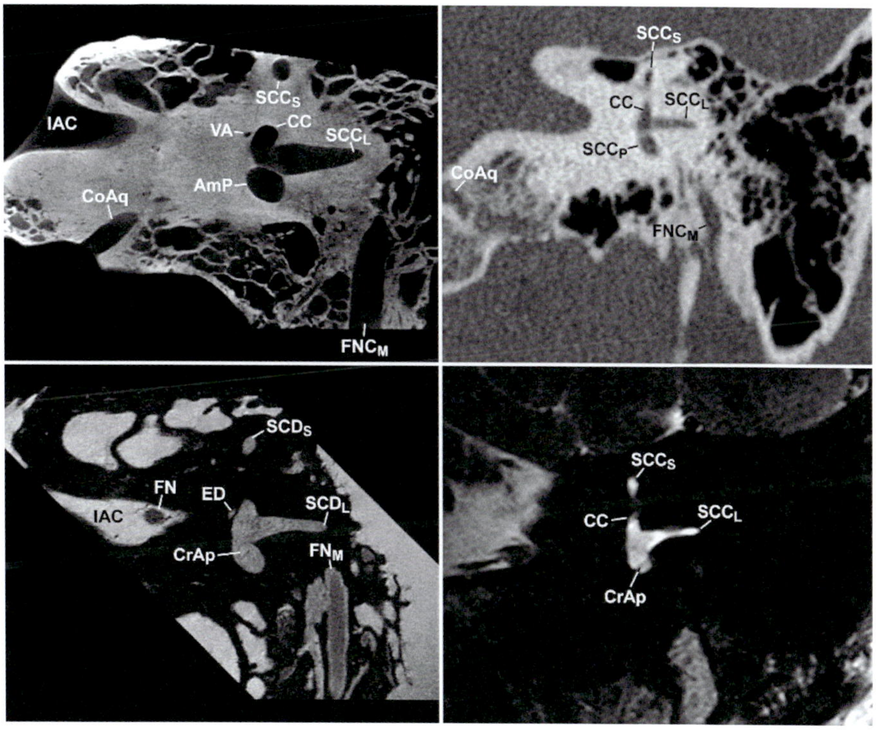
IAC
SCC$_S$
VA
CC
SCC$_L$
AmP
CoAq
FNC$_M$
SCC$_P$
SCD$_S$
FN
ED
SCD$_L$
CrAp
FN$_M$

Fig. 33

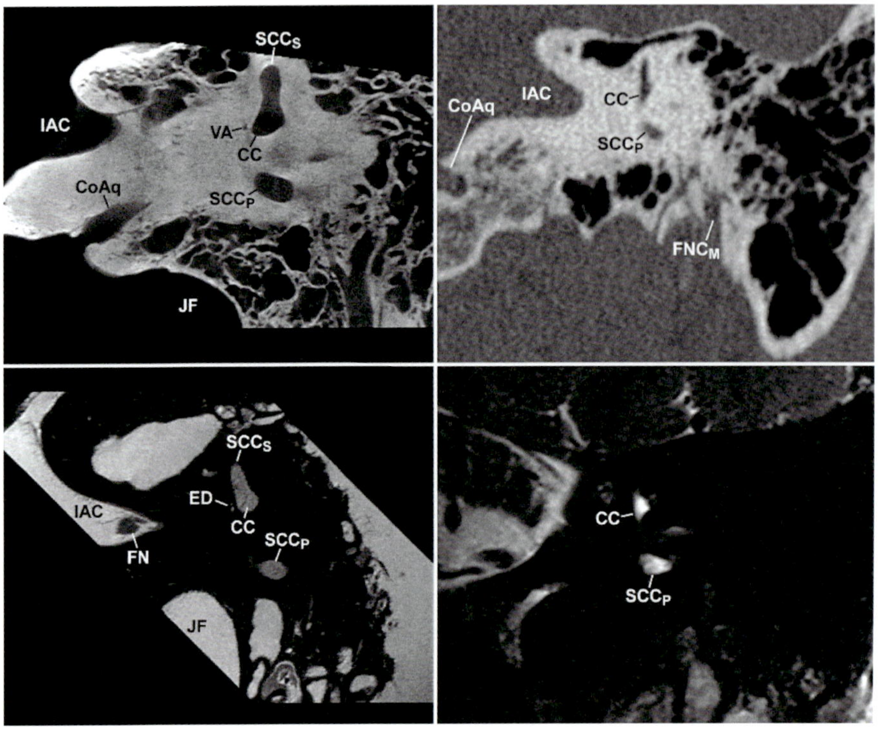
SCCS
IAC
VA
CC
CoAq
SCCP
JF
IAC
CoAq
CC
SCCP
FNCM
SCCS
ED
IAC
CC
SCCP
FN
JF
CC
SCCP

Fig. 34

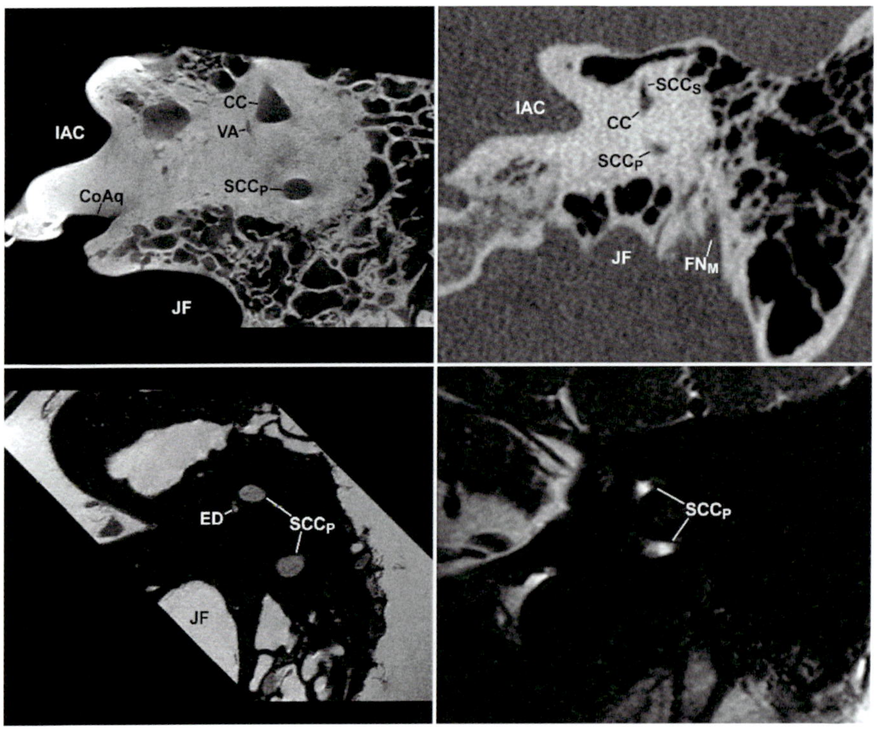
IAC
CC
VA
CoAq
SCCP
JF
SCCS
IAC
CC
SCCP
JF
FNM
ED
SCCP
JF
SCCP

Fig. 35

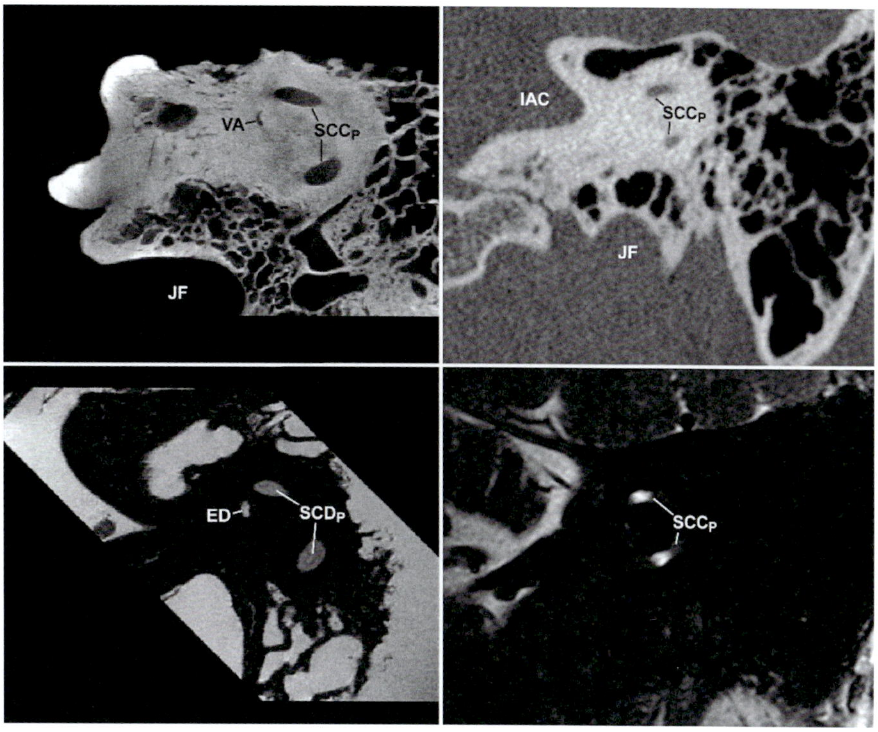
VA
SCCP
JF
IAC
SCCP
JF
ED
SCDP
SCCP

Fig. 36

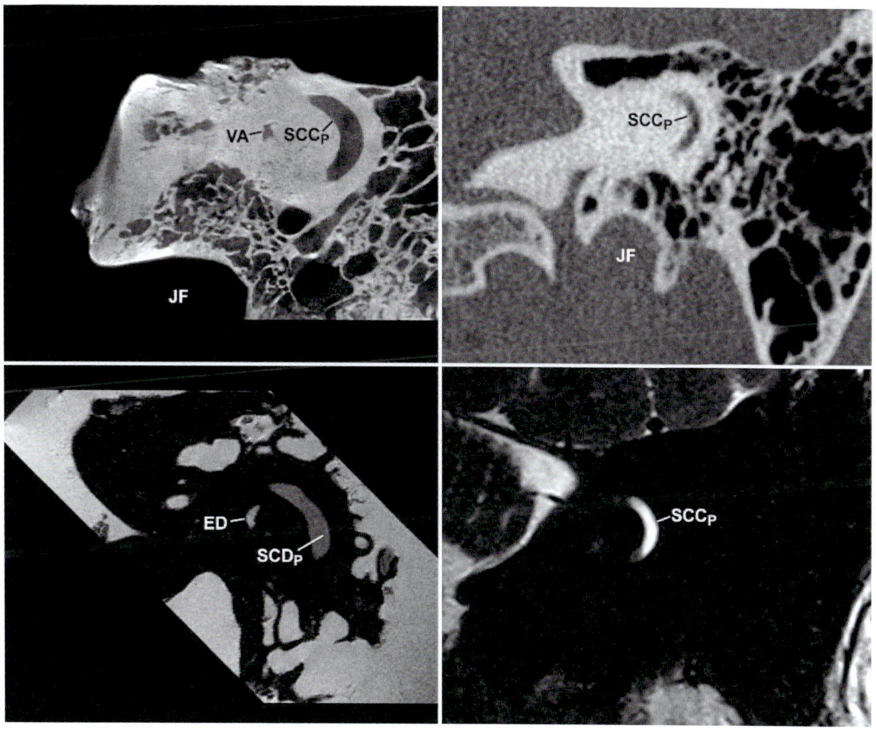
VA
SCCP
JF
SCCP
JF
ED
SCDP
SCCP

Fig. 37

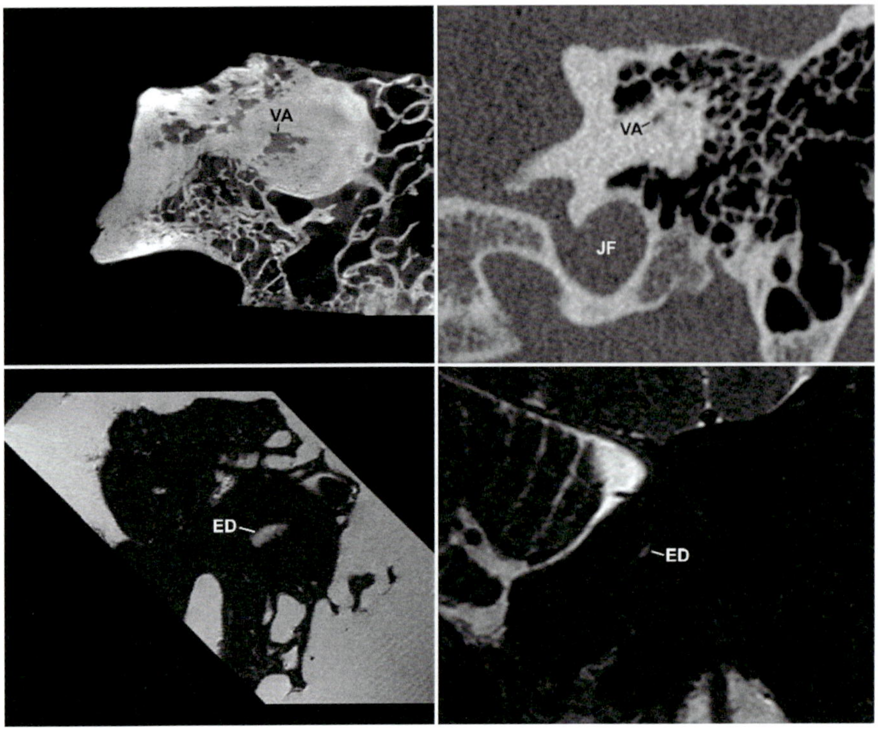

Fig. 38

Pöschl Plane (Short Axis Plane of the Temporal Bone)

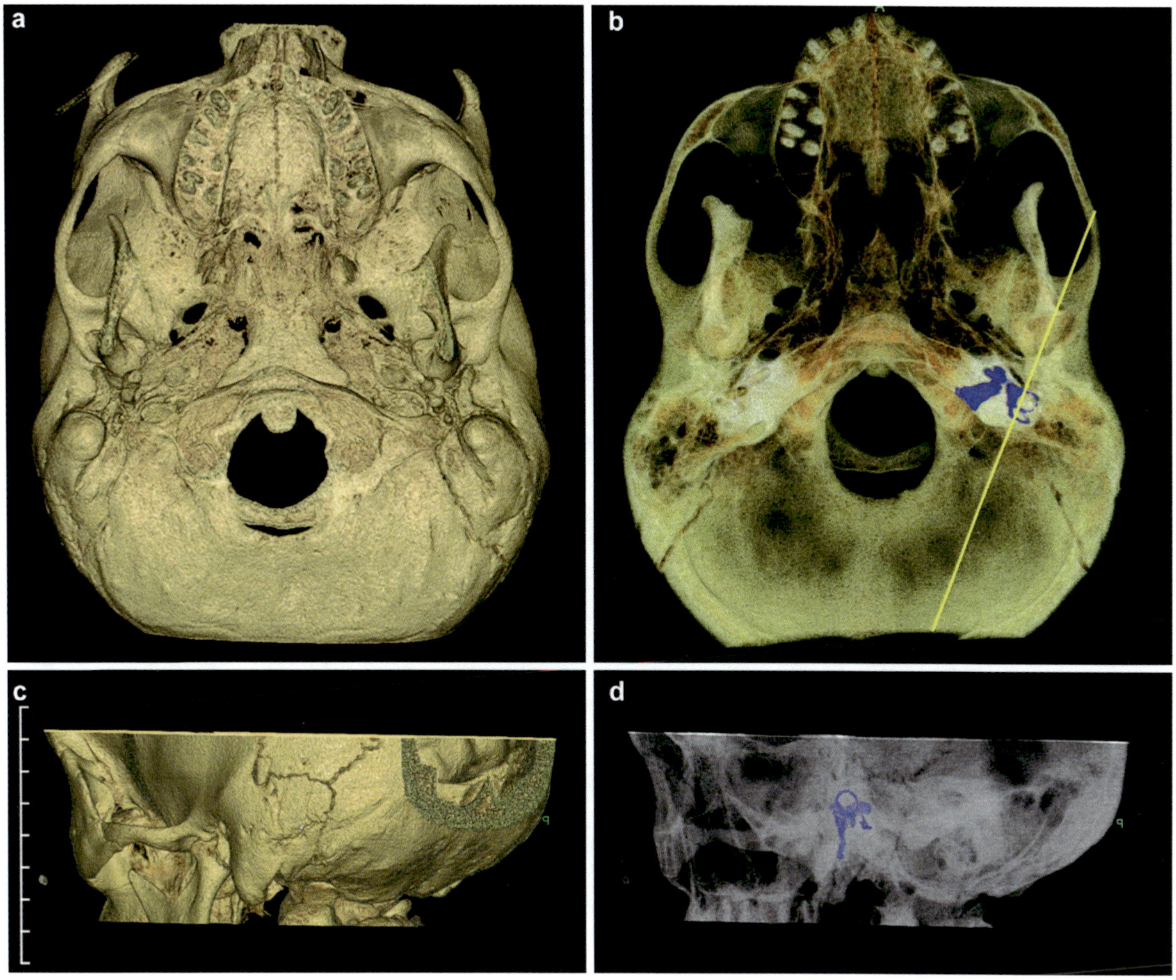

Fig. 39 Pöschl plane of section through the left temporal bone. (**a**) Inferior view of 3D surface-rendered reconstruction from MDCT volume. (**b**) Maximum intensity projection with color-segmented labyrinth showing orientation of the superior semicircular canal. Yellow line indicates the plane of section parallel to the superior semicircular canal. (**c**) Posterolateral oblique view of 3D surface-rendered reconstruction from MDCT volume oriented in the Pöschl plane. (**d**) Maximum intensity projection demonstrating orientation of the labyrinth in the Pöschl plane to include the course of the facial nerve canal

The following serial images in the Pöschl plane are presented from lateral to medial to include microCT (*upper left*), MDCT (*upper right*), microMR (*lower left*), and 3T MR (*lower right*).

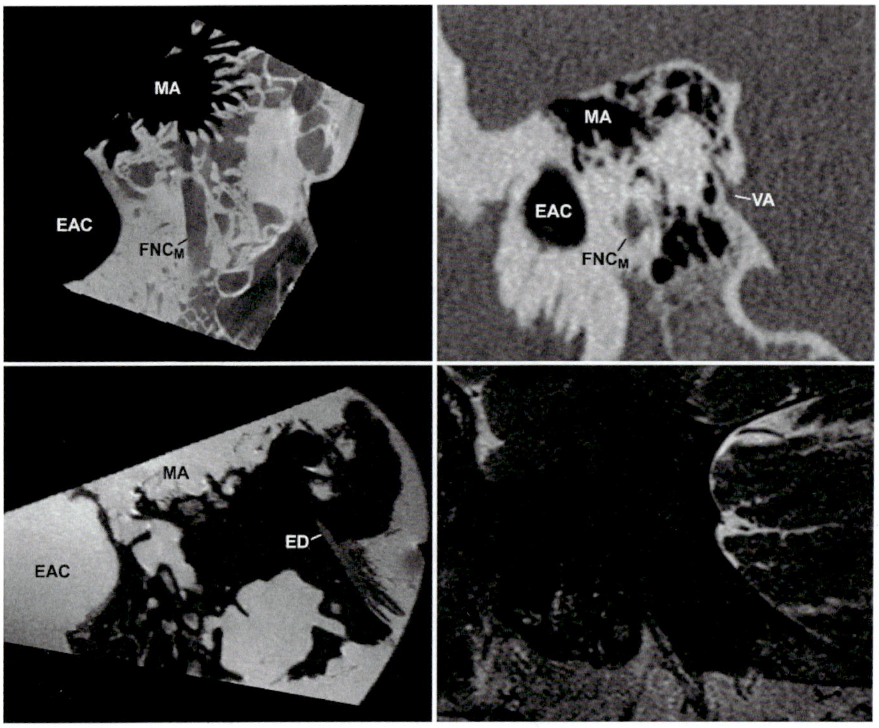

Fig. 40

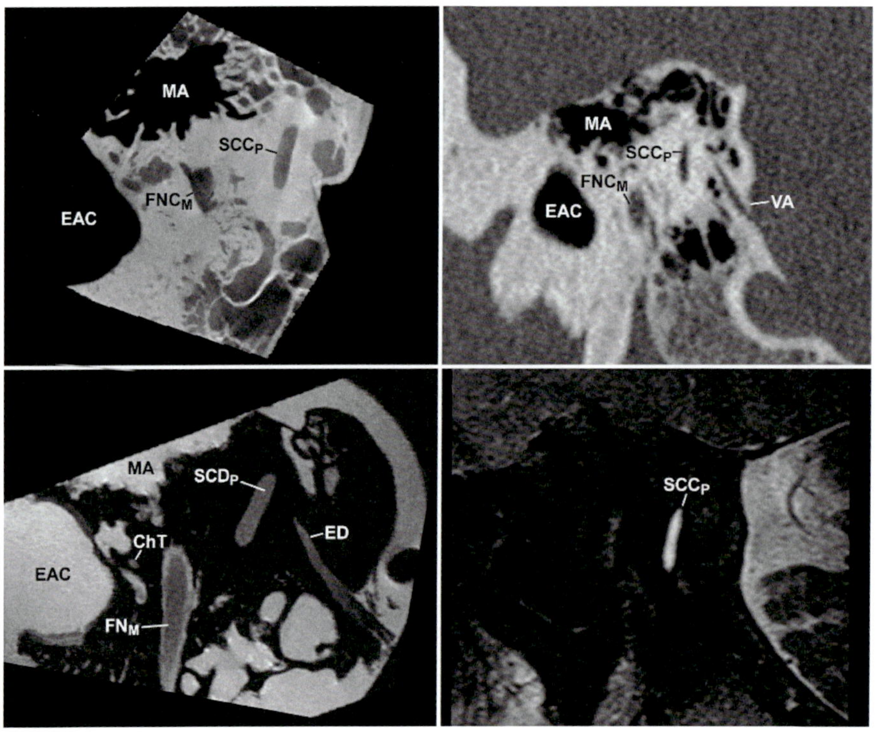

Fig. 41

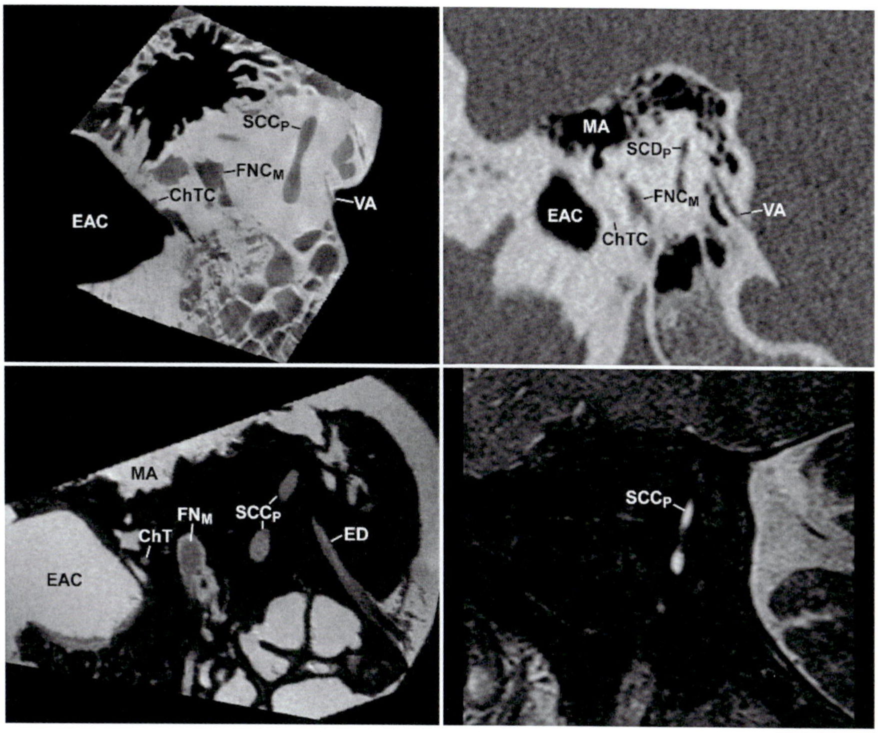

SCC_P
FNC_M
ChTC
VA
EAC
MA
SCD_P
FNC_M
ChTC
VA
EAC
MA
FN_M
SCC_P
ChT
ED
EAC
SCC_P

Fig. 42

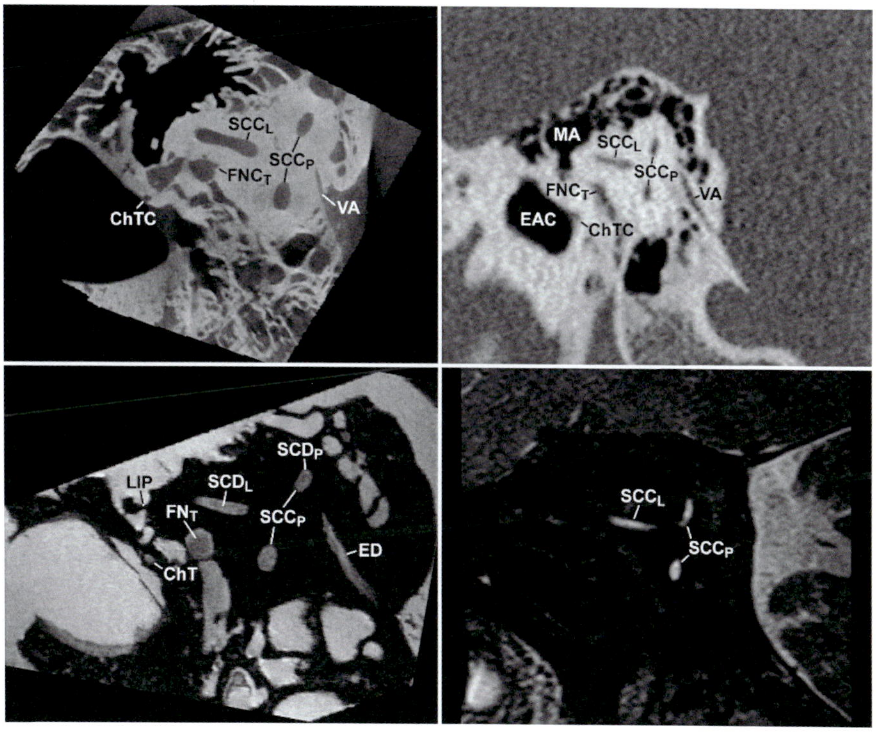

SCC_L
SCC_P
FNC_T
VA
ChTC
MA
SCC_L
SCC_P
FNC_T
VA
EAC
ChTC
SCD_P
LIP
SCD_L
FN_T
SCC_P
ED
ChT
SCC_L
SCC_P

Fig. 43

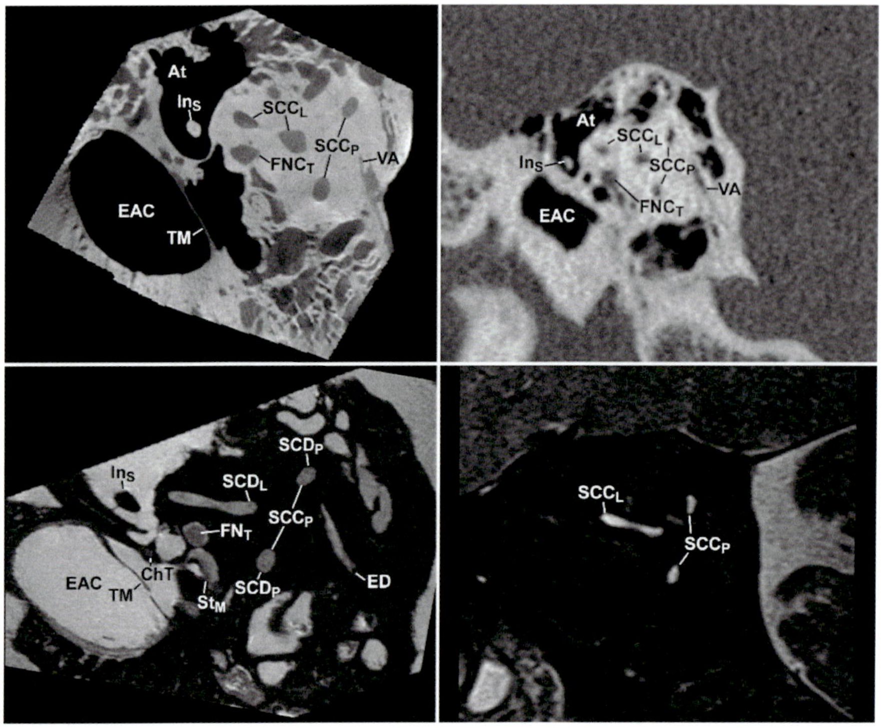
At
Ins
SCCL
SCCP
FNCT
VA
EAC
TM
At
SCCL
Ins
SCCP
VA
EAC
FNCT
SCDP
Ins
SCDL
SCCP
FNT
EAC
ChT
TM
StM
SCDP
ED
SCCL
SCCP

Fig. 44

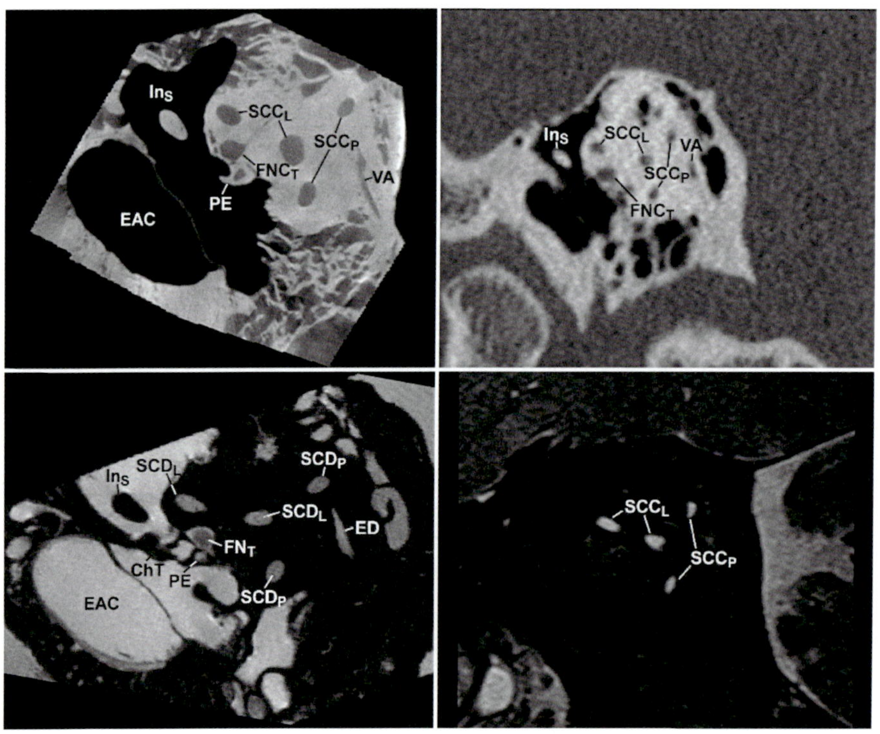
Ins
SCCL
SCCP
FNCT
VA
PE
EAC
Ins
SCCL
VA
SCCP
FNCT
SCDP
Ins
SCDL
SCDL
ED
FNT
ChT
PE
EAC
SCDP
SCCL
SCCP

Fig. 45

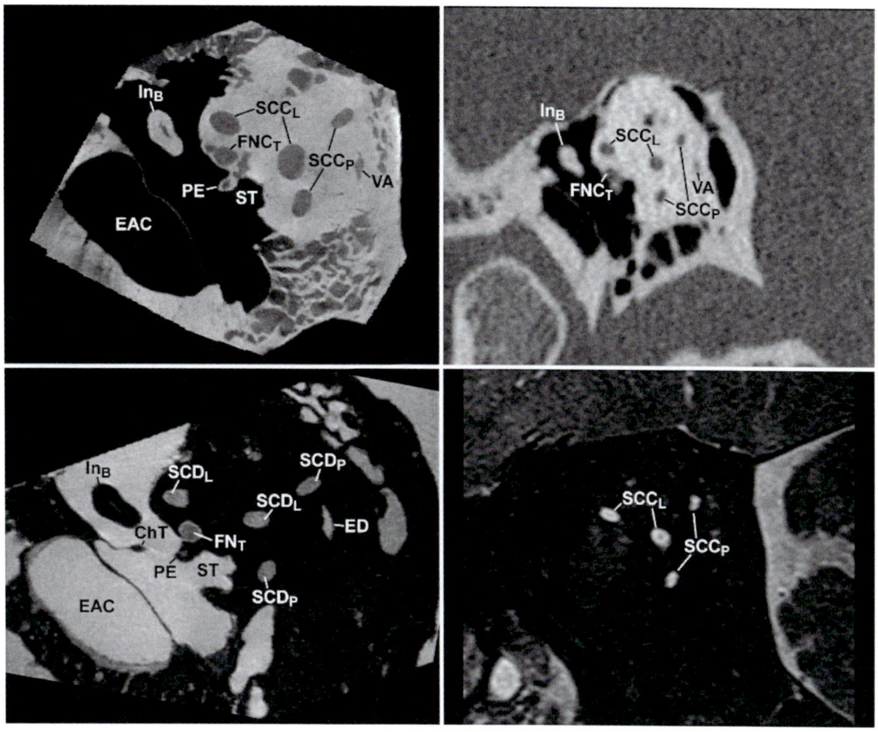
InB
SCCL
FNCT
SCCP
VA
PE
ST
EAC
InB
SCCL
FNCT
VA
SCCP
InB
SCDL
SCDP
SCDL
ED
ChT
FNT
PE
ST
SCDP
EAC
SCCL
SCCP

Fig. 46

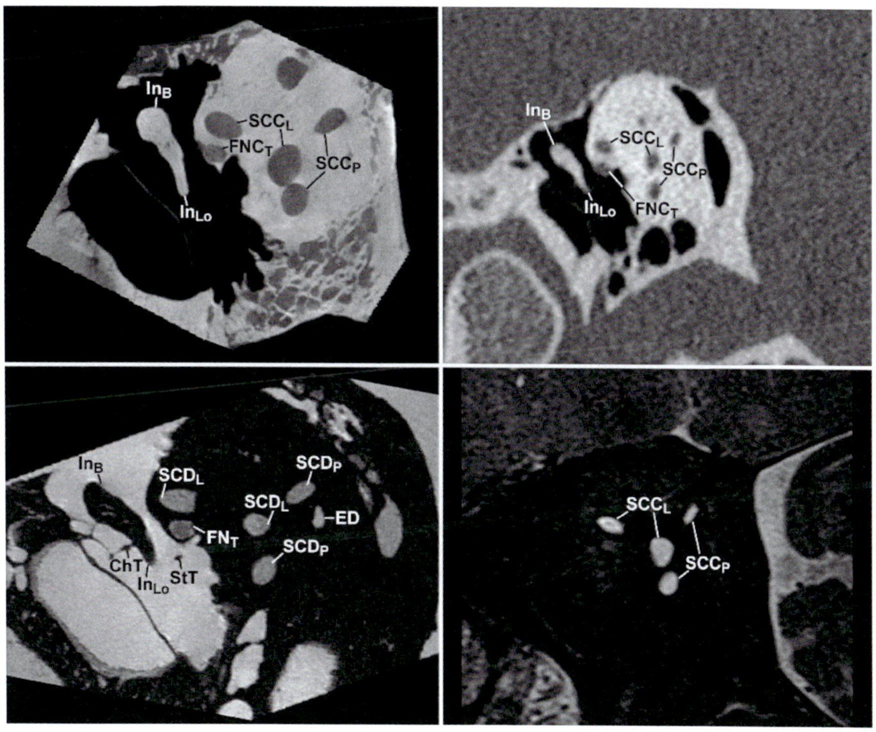
InB
SCCL
FNCT
SCCP
InLo
InB
SCCL
SCCP
InLo
FNCT
InB
SCDL
SCDP
SCDL
ED
FNT
SCDP
ChT
InLo
StT
SCCL
SCCP

Fig. 47

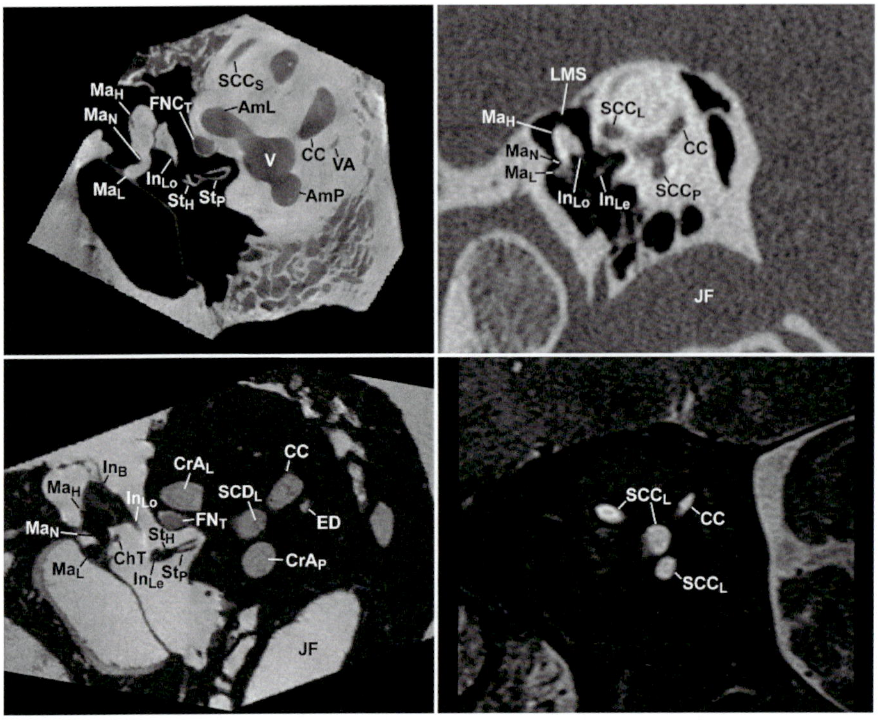
SCC_S
Ma_H
Ma_N
FNC_T
AmL
V
CC
VA
Ma_L
In_{Lo}
St_H
St_P
AmP
LMS
SCC_L
Ma_H
Ma_N
Ma_L
CC
In_{Lo}
In_{Le}
SCC_P
JF
In_B
Ma_H
In_{Lo}
CrA_L
SCD_L
CC
FN_T
ED
Ma_N
St_H
ChT
CrA_P
Ma_L
In_{Le}
St_P
JF
SCC_L
CC
SCC_L

Fig. 48

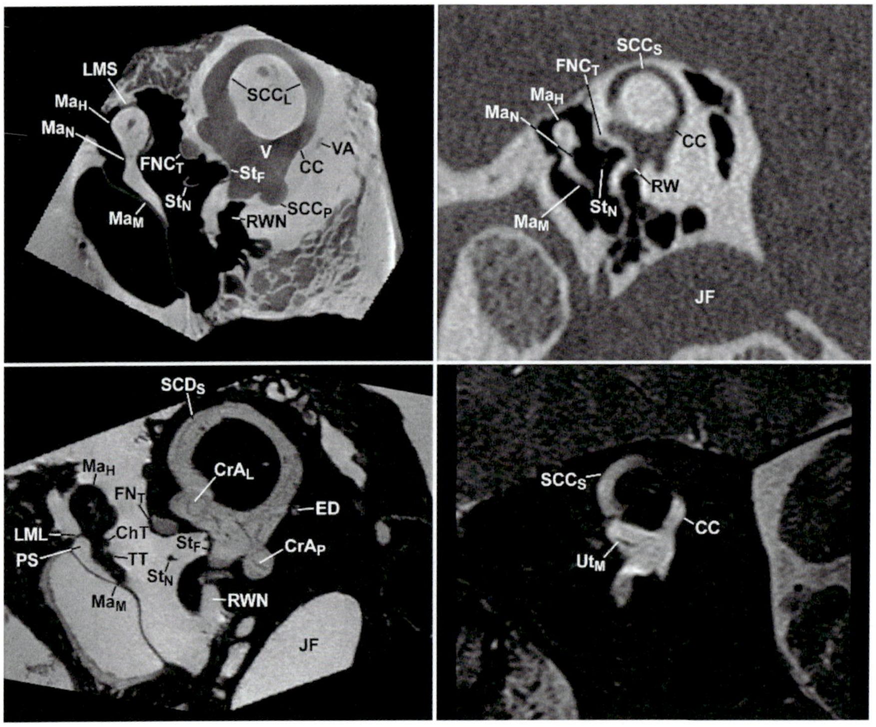
LMS
Ma_H
Ma_N
SCC_L
V
VA
FNC_T
St_F
CC
St_N
Ma_M
RWN
SCC_P
SCC_S
FNC_T
Ma_H
Ma_N
CC
RW
St_N
Ma_M
JF
SCD_S
Ma_H
CrA_L
FN_T
ED
LML
ChT
St_F
CrA_P
PS
TT
St_N
Ma_M
RWN
JF
SCC_S
CC
Ut_M

Fig. 49

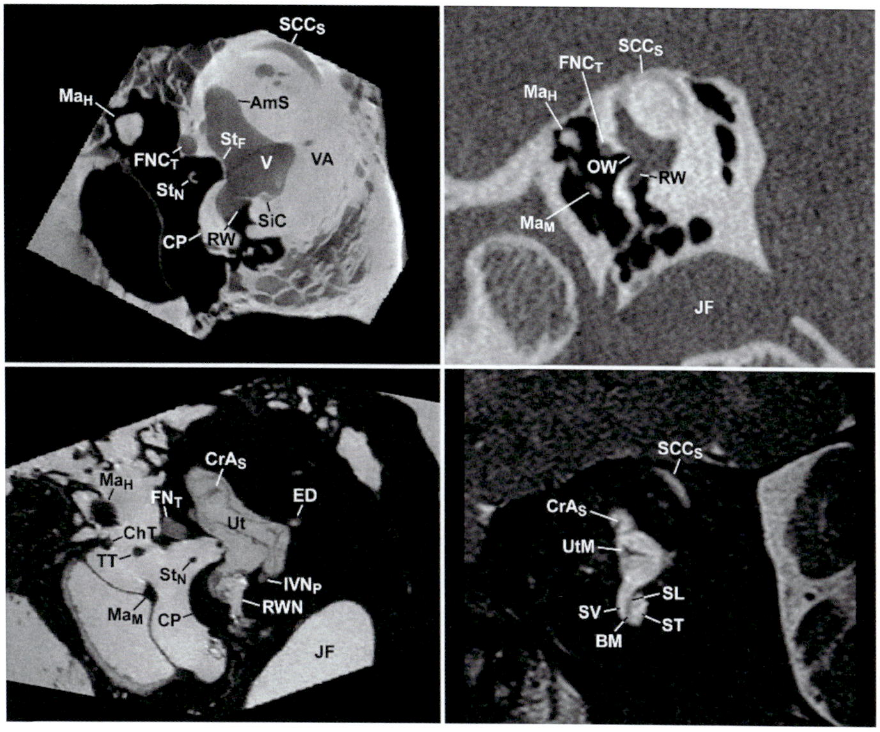
SCC_S
Ma_H
AmS
St_F
FNC_T
V
VA
St_N
SiC
CP
RW
SCC_S
FNC_T
Ma_H
OW
RW
Ma_M
JF
CrA_S
Ma_H
FN_T
ED
Ut
ChT
TT
St_N
IVN_P
RWN
Ma_M
CP
JF
SCC_S
CrA_S
UtM
SL
SV
ST
BM

Fig. 50

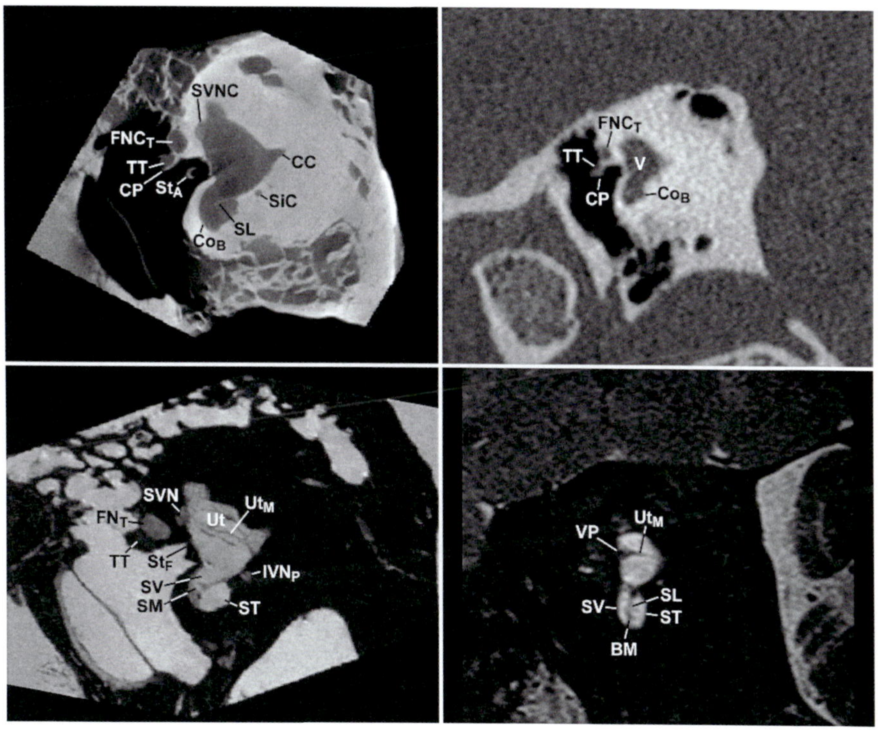
SVNC
FNC_T
CC
TT
CP
St_A
SiC
SL
Co_B
FNC_T
TT
V
CP
Co_B
SVN
Ut_M
FN_T
Ut
TT
St_F
IVN_P
SV
SM
ST
Ut_M
VP
SL
SV
ST
BM

Fig. 51

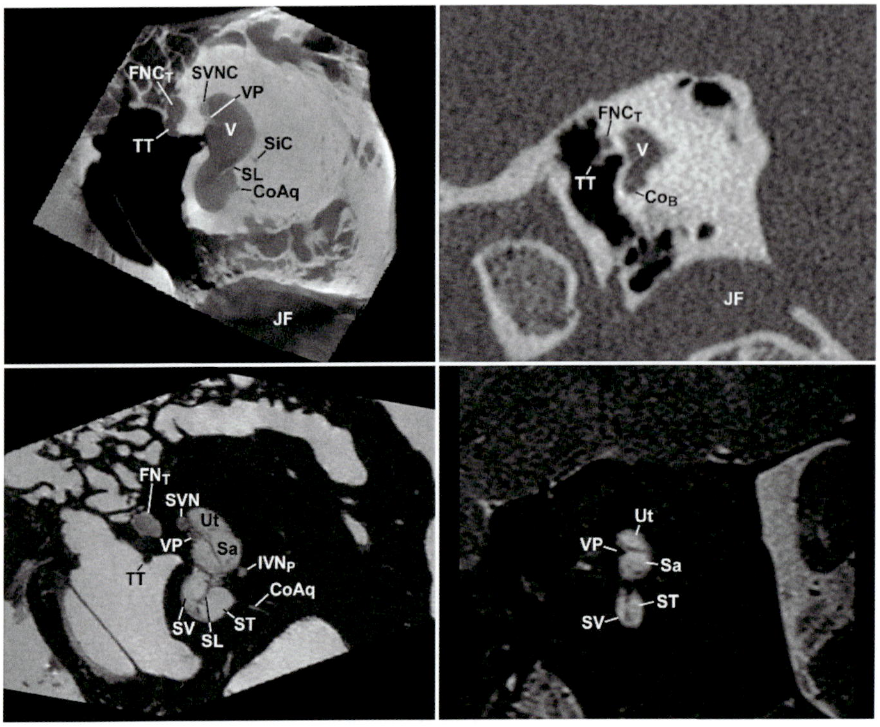
FNC$_{T}$
SVNC
VP
V
TT
SiC
SL
CoAq
JF
FNC$_{T}$
V
TT
Co$_{B}$
JF
FN$_{T}$
SVN
Ut
VP
Sa
IVN$_{P}$
TT
CoAq
SV
SL
ST
Ut
VP
Sa
ST
SV

Fig. 52

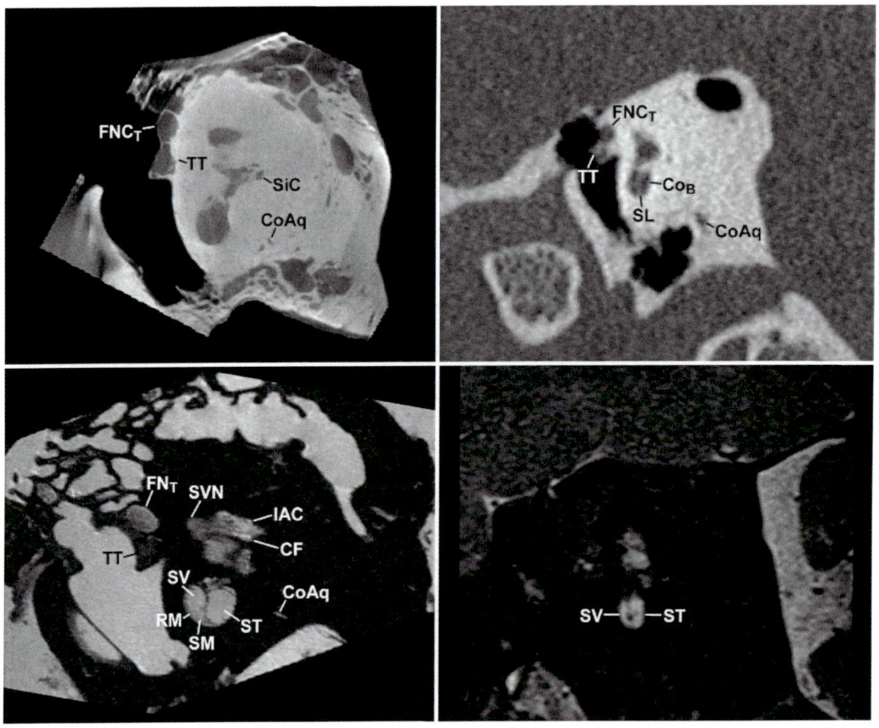
FNC$_{T}$
TT
SiC
CoAq
FNC$_{T}$
TT
Co$_{B}$
SL
CoAq
FN$_{T}$
SVN
IAC
CF
TT
SV
CoAq
RM
ST
SM
SV
ST

Fig. 53

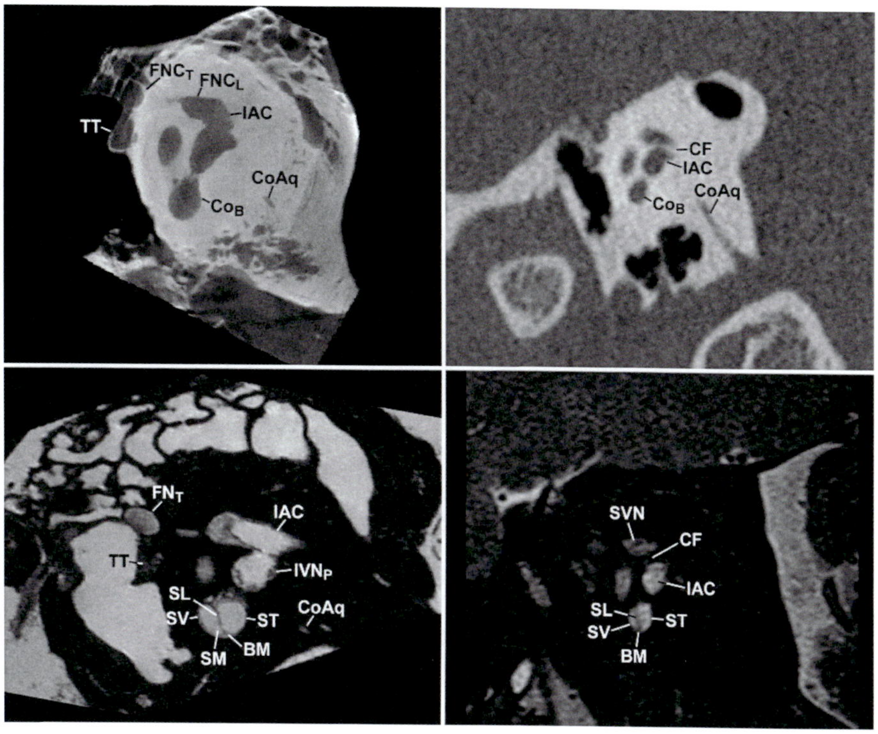
FNC_T
FNC_L
IAC
TT
CoAq
Co_B
CF
IAC
Co_B
CoAq
FN_T
IAC
TT
IVN_P
SL
SV
ST
CoAq
BM
SM
SVN
CF
IAC
SL
ST
SV
BM

Fig. 54

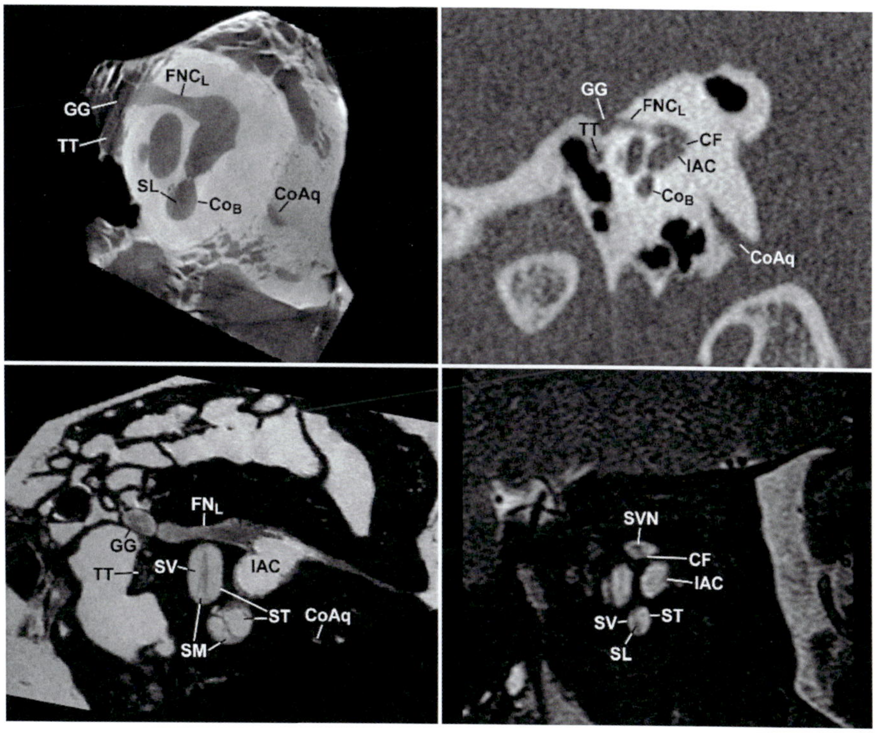
FNC_L
GG
TT
SL
Co_B
CoAq
GG
FNC_L
TT
CF
IAC
Co_B
CoAq
FN_L
GG
TT
SV
IAC
ST
CoAq
SM
SVN
CF
IAC
SV
ST
SL

Fig. 55

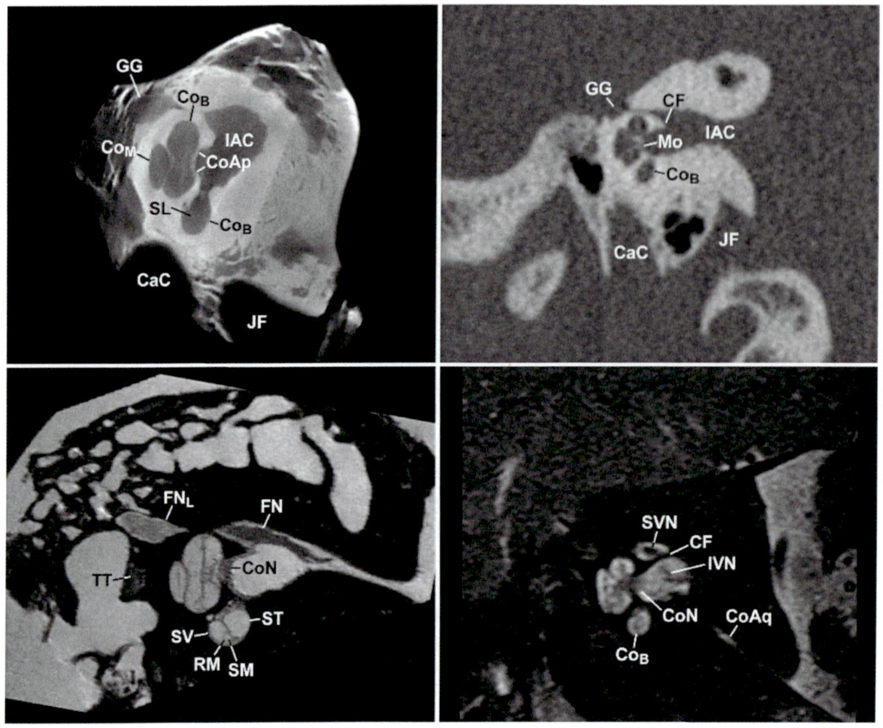
GG
CoB
IAC
CoM
CoAp
SL
CoB
CaC
JF
GG
CF
Mo
IAC
CoB
CaC
JF
FNL
FN
TT
CoN
ST
SV
RM
SM
SVN
CF
IVN
CoN
CoAq
CoB

Fig. 56

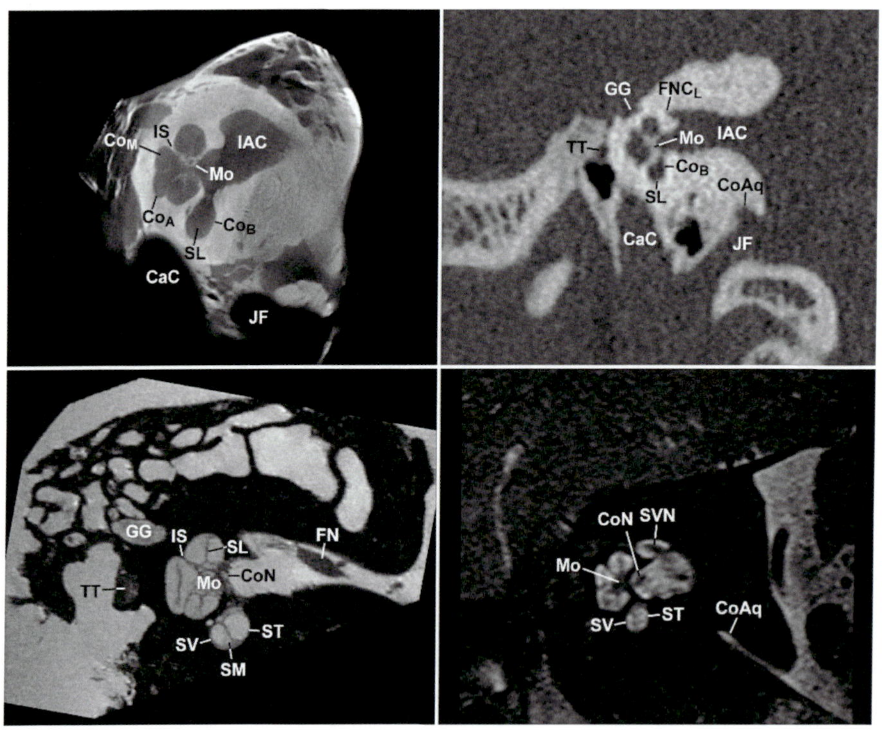
CoM
IS
IAC
Mo
CoA
CoB
SL
CaC
JF
GG
FNCL
TT
Mo
IAC
CoB
SL
CoAq
CaC
JF
GG
IS
SL
FN
TT
Mo
CoN
SV
ST
SM
CoN
SVN
Mo
SV
ST
CoAq

Fig. 57

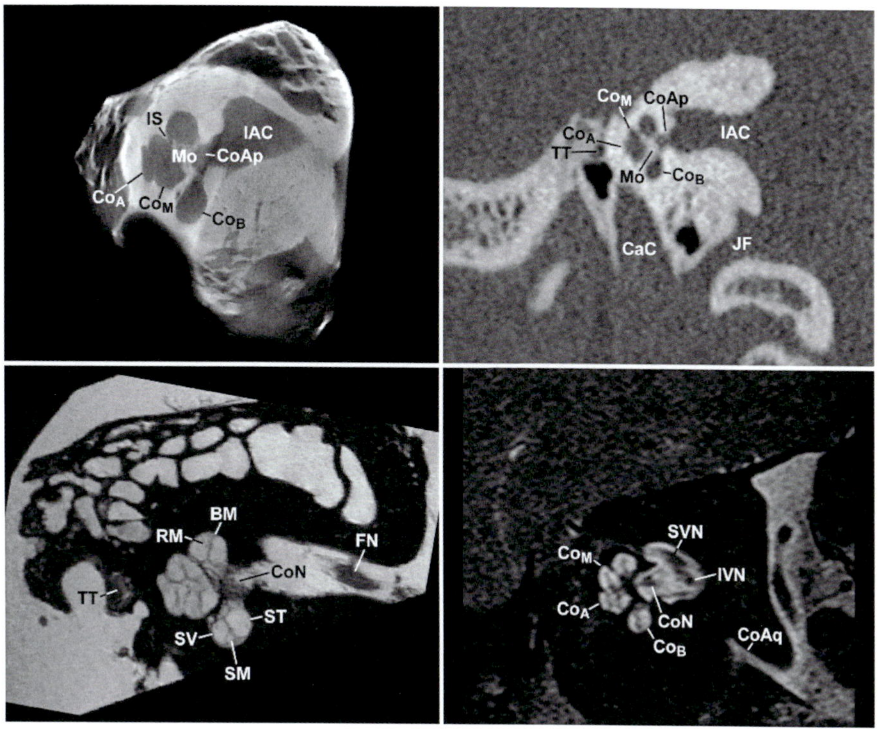
IS
IAC
Mo
CoAp
CoA
CoM
CoB
CoM
CoAp
CoA
TT
IAC
Mo
CoB
CaC
JF
BM
RM
FN
CoN
TT
ST
SV
SM
SVN
CoM
IVN
CoA
CoN
CoB
CoAq

Fig. 58

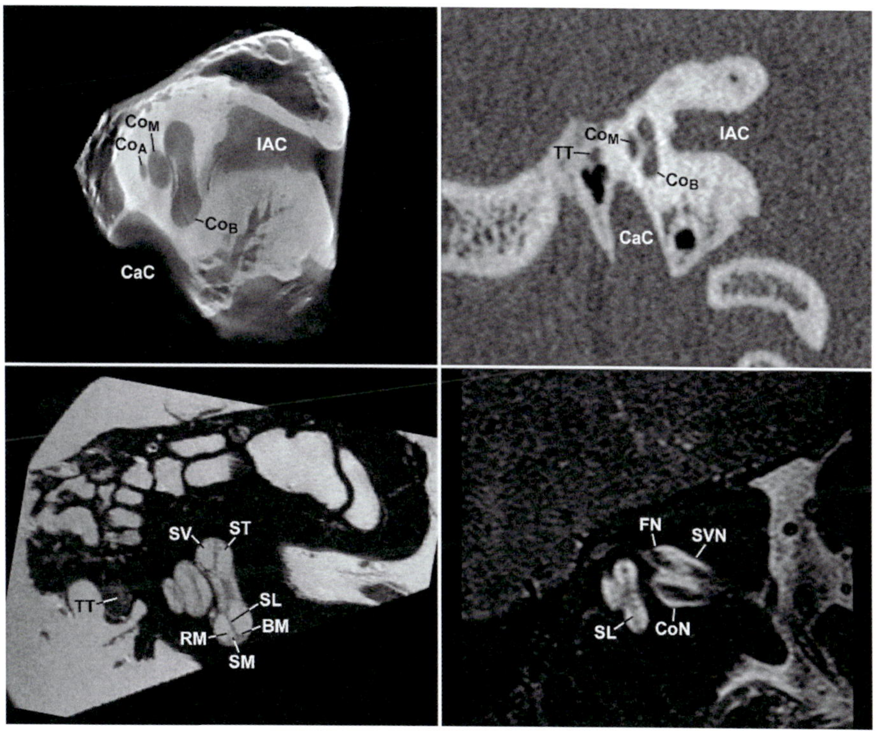
CoM
CoA
IAC
CoB
CaC
CoM
TT
IAC
CoB
CaC
SV
ST
TT
SL
RM
BM
SM
FN
SVN
SL
CoN

Fig. 59

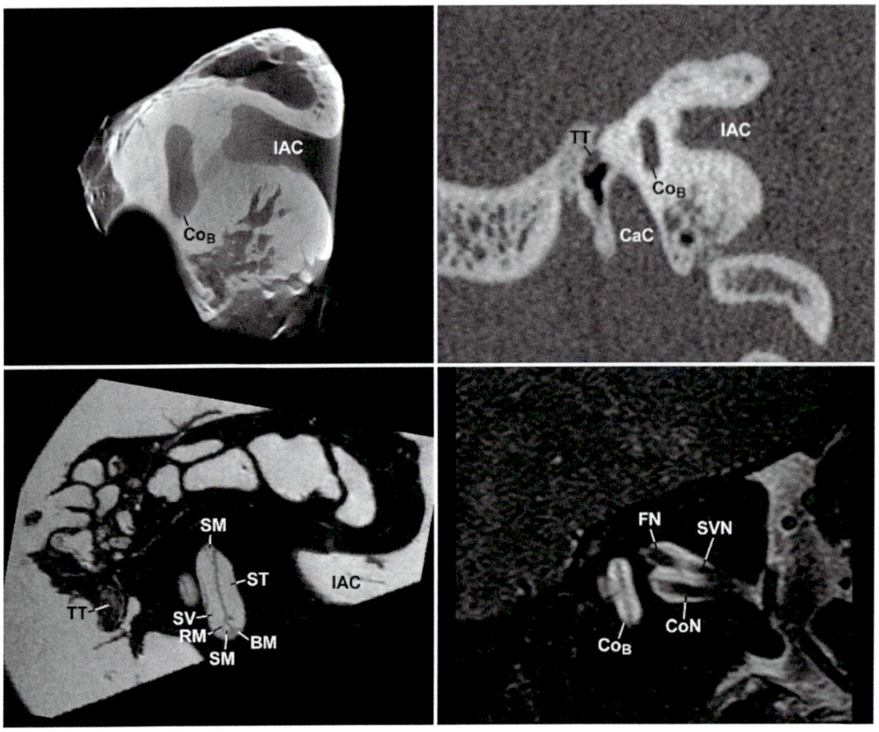
IAC
CoB
TT
IAC
CoB
CaC
SM
ST
IAC
TT
SV
RM
SM
BM
FN
SVN
CoB
CoN

Fig. 60

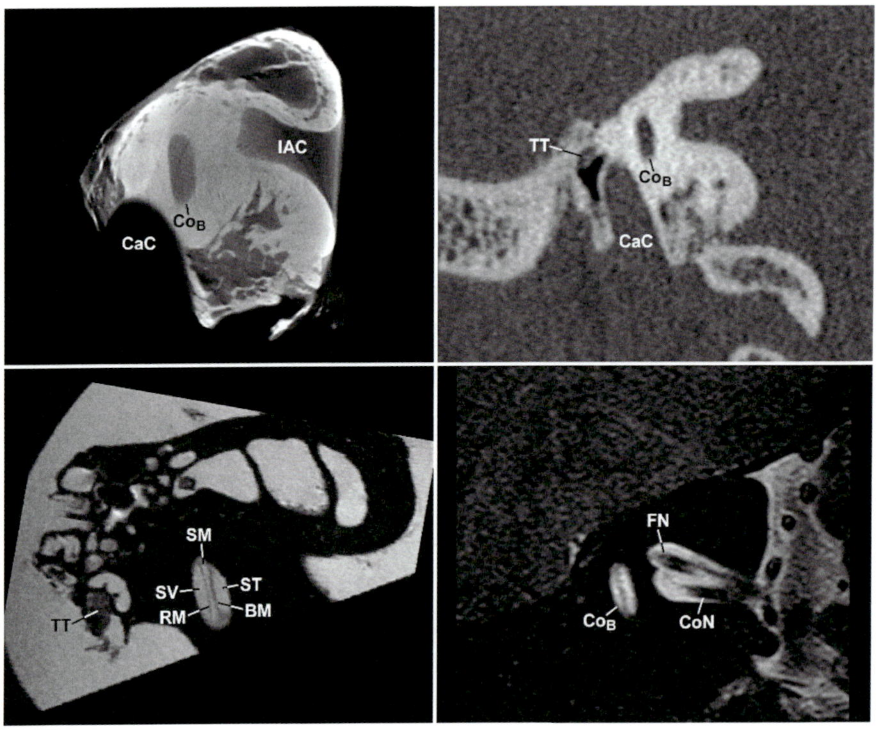
IAC
CoB
CaC
TT
CoB
CaC
SM
SV
ST
TT
RM
BM
FN
CoB
CoN

Fig. 61

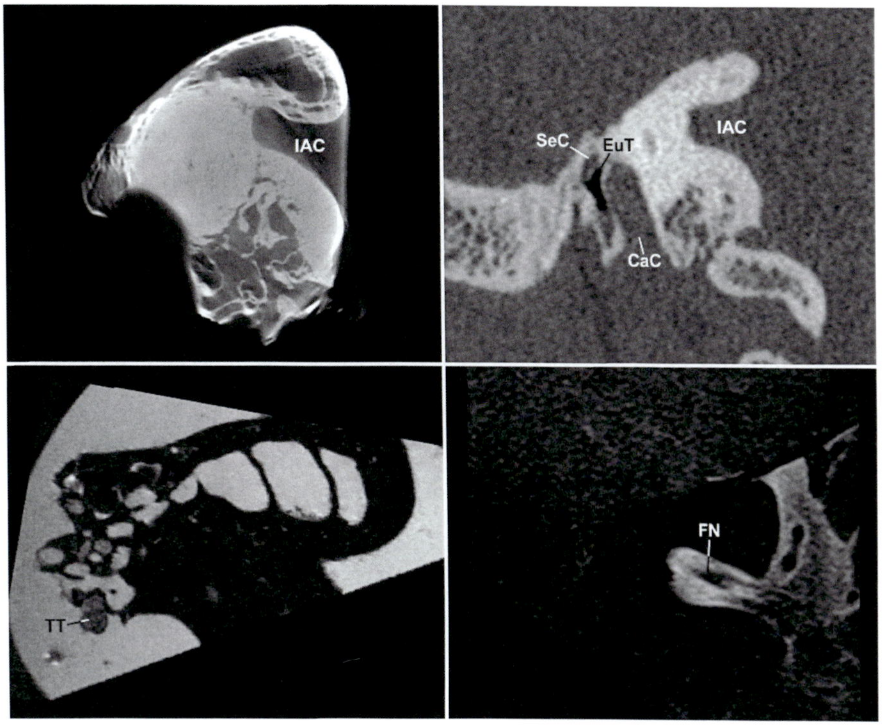

Fig. 62

Stenvers Plane (Long Axis Plane of the Temporal Bone)

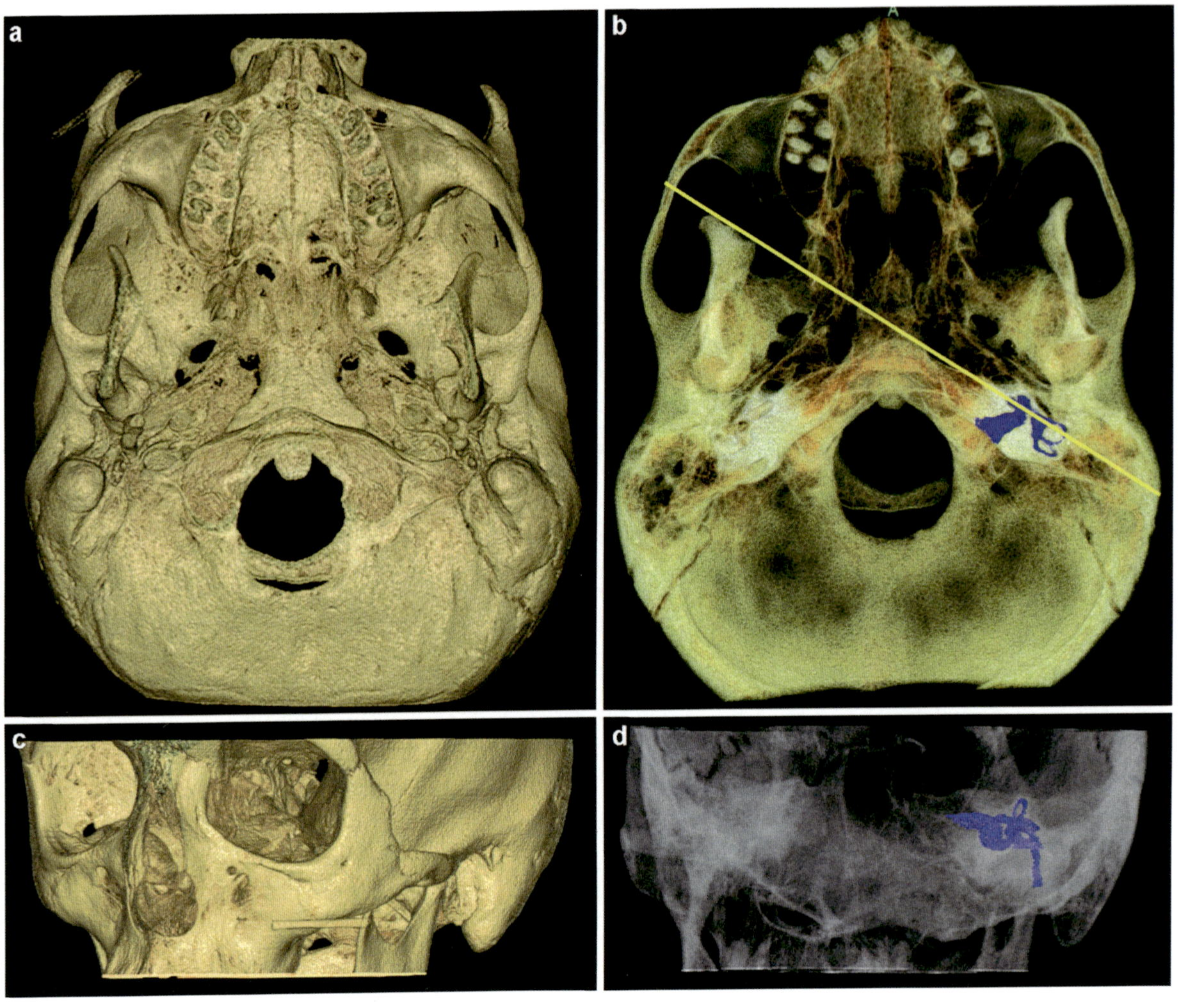

Fig. 63 Stenvers plane of section through the left temporal bone. (**a**) Inferior view of 3D surface-rendered reconstruction from MDCT volume. (**b**) Maximum intensity projection with color-segmented labyrinth showing orientation of the superior semicircular canal. *Yellow line* indicates the plane of section perpendicular to the superior semicircular canal. (**c**) Left anterolalateral oblique view of 3D surface-rendered reconstruction from MDCT volume oriented in the Stenvers plane of section. (**d**) Maximum intensity projection demonstrating orientation of the labyrinth in the Stenvers plane to include the course of the facial nerve canal

The following serial images in the Stenvers plane are presented from anterior to posterior to include microCT (*upper left*), MDCT (*upper right*), microMR (*lower left*), and 3T MR (*lower right*).

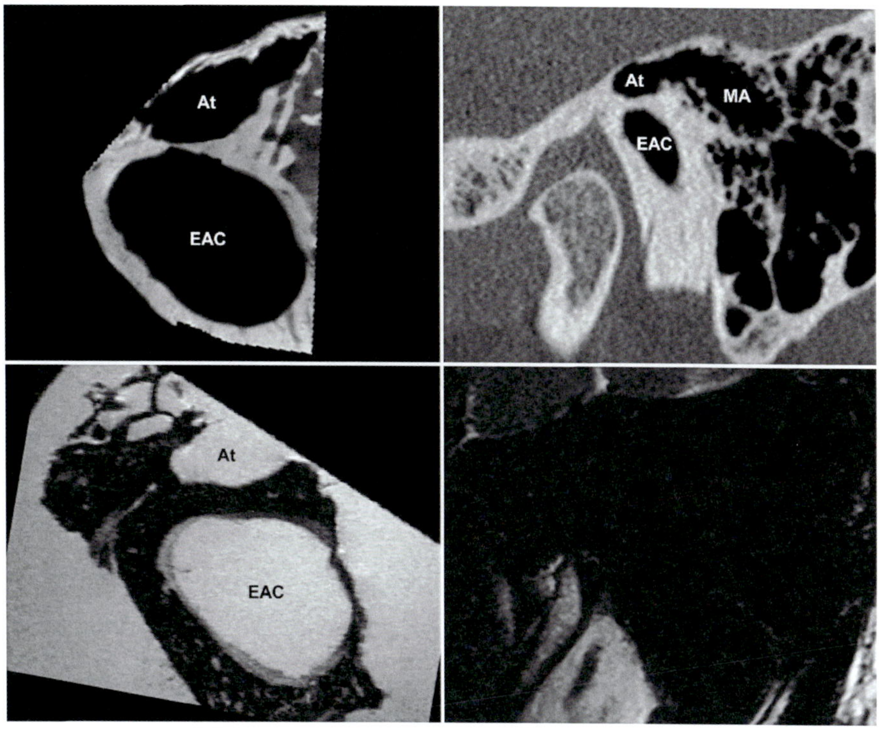

Fig. 64

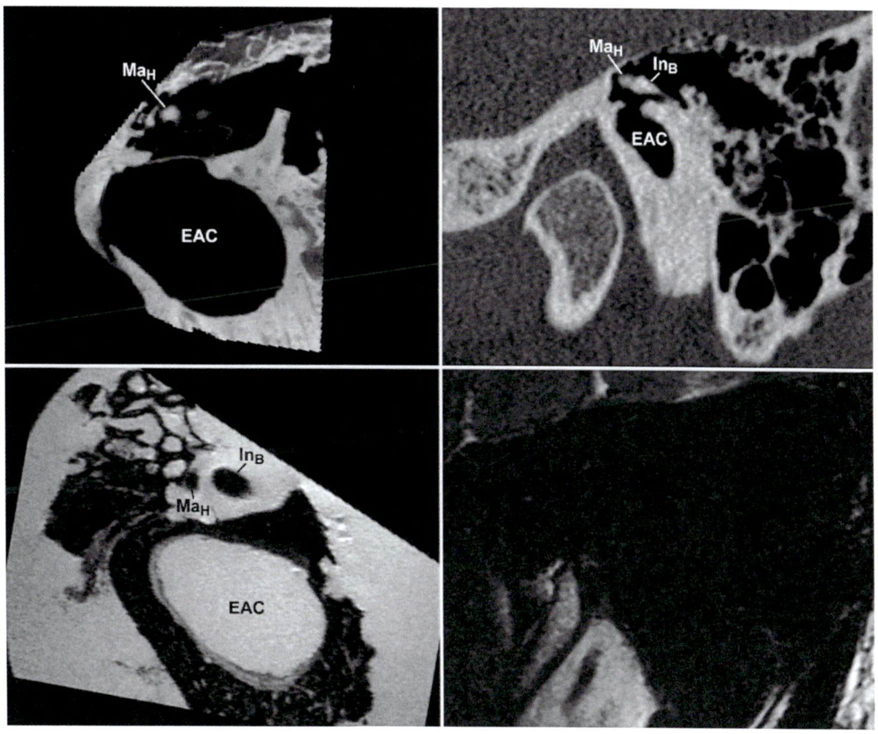

Fig. 65

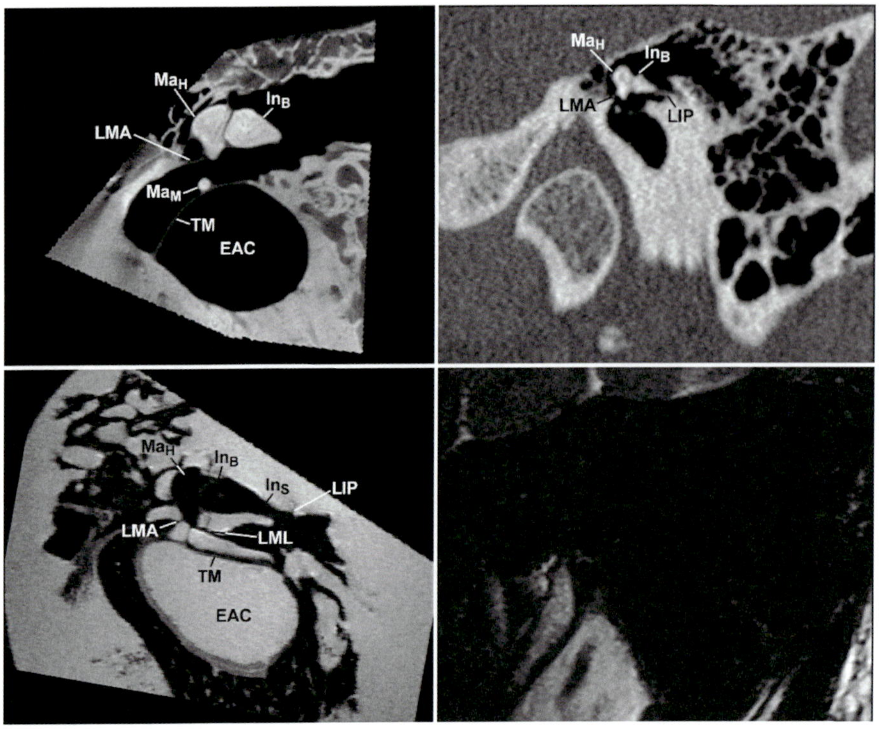
MaH
InB
LMA
MaM
TM
EAC
MaH
InB
LMA
LIP
MaH
InB
InS
LIP
LMA
LML
TM
EAC
Fig. 66

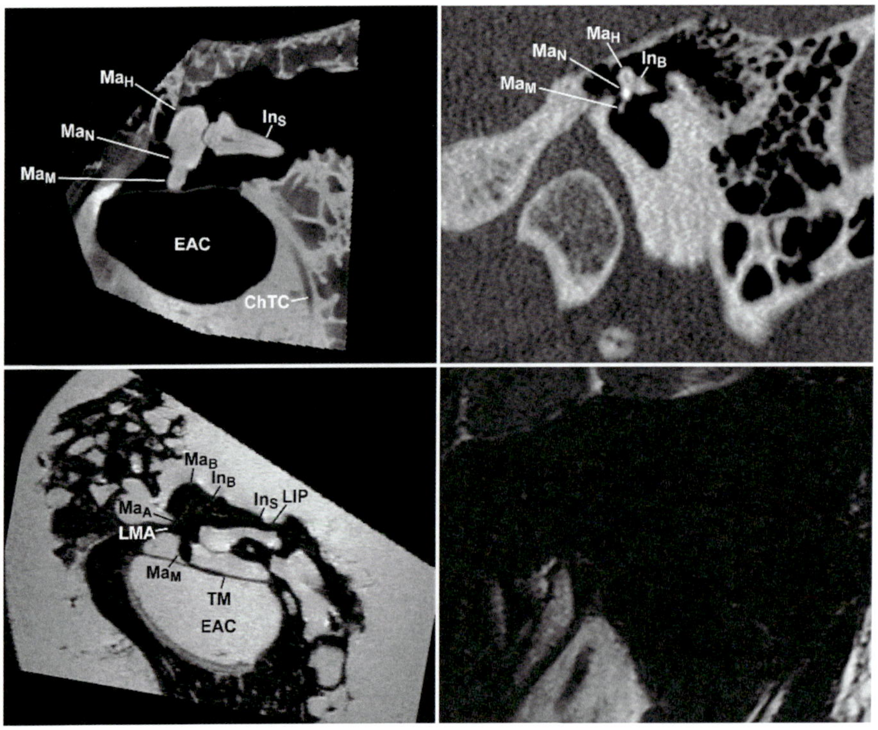
MaH
MaN
InS
MaM
EAC
ChTC
MaH
MaN
InB
MaM
MaB
InB
MaA
InS
LIP
LMA
MaM
TM
EAC
Fig. 67

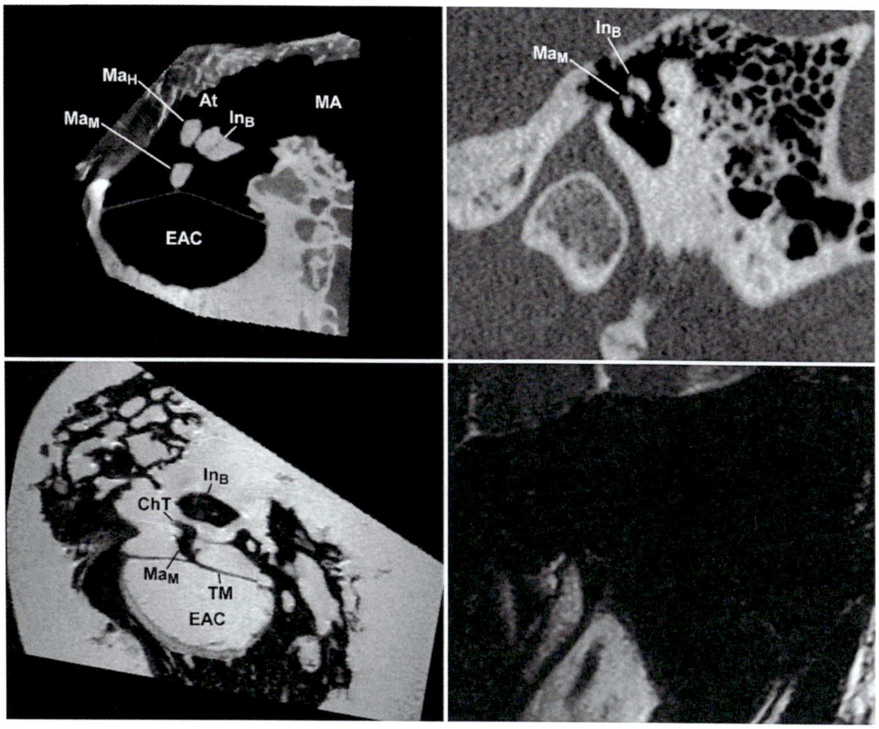
MaH
At
InB
MA
MaM
EAC
InB
MaM
InB
ChT
MaM
TM
EAC

Fig. 68

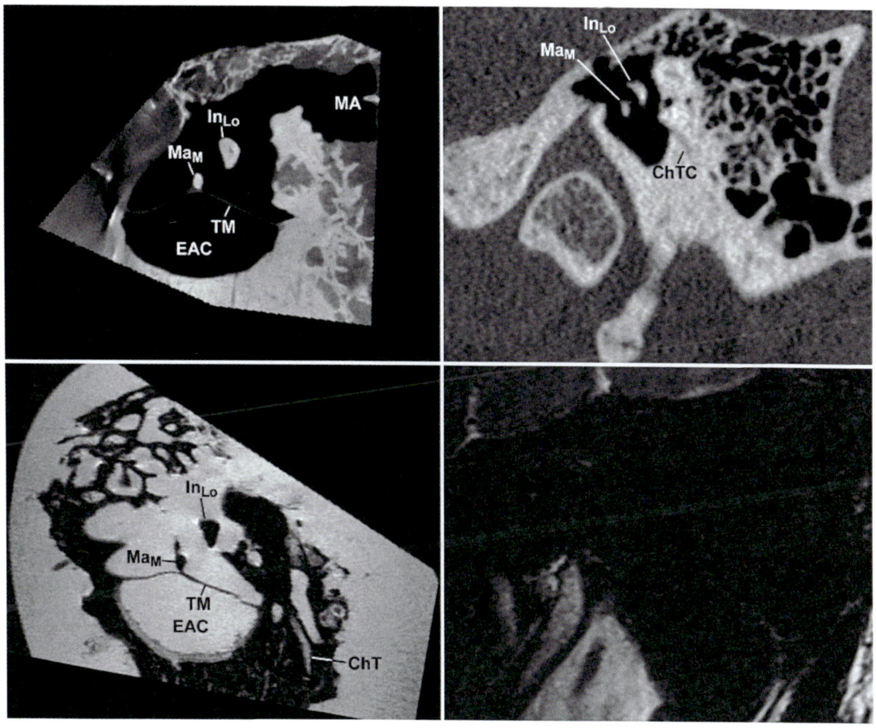
MA
InLo
MaM
TM
EAC
InLo
MaM
ChTC
InLo
MaM
TM
EAC
ChT

Fig. 69

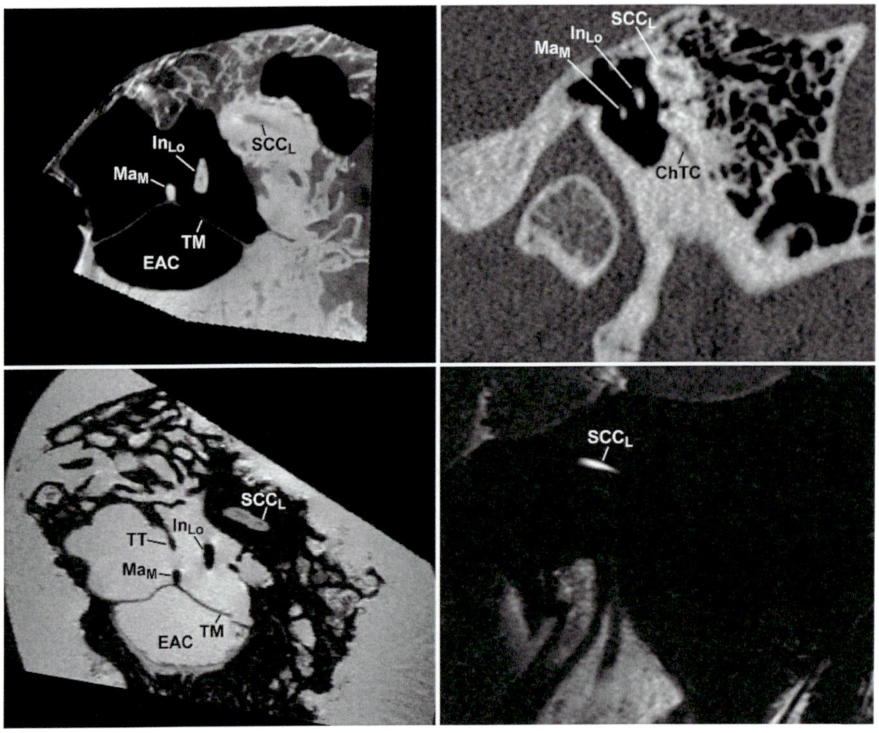
In_{Lo}
SCC_L
Ma_M
TM
EAC
Ma_M
ChTC
SCC_L
TT
EAC

Fig. 70

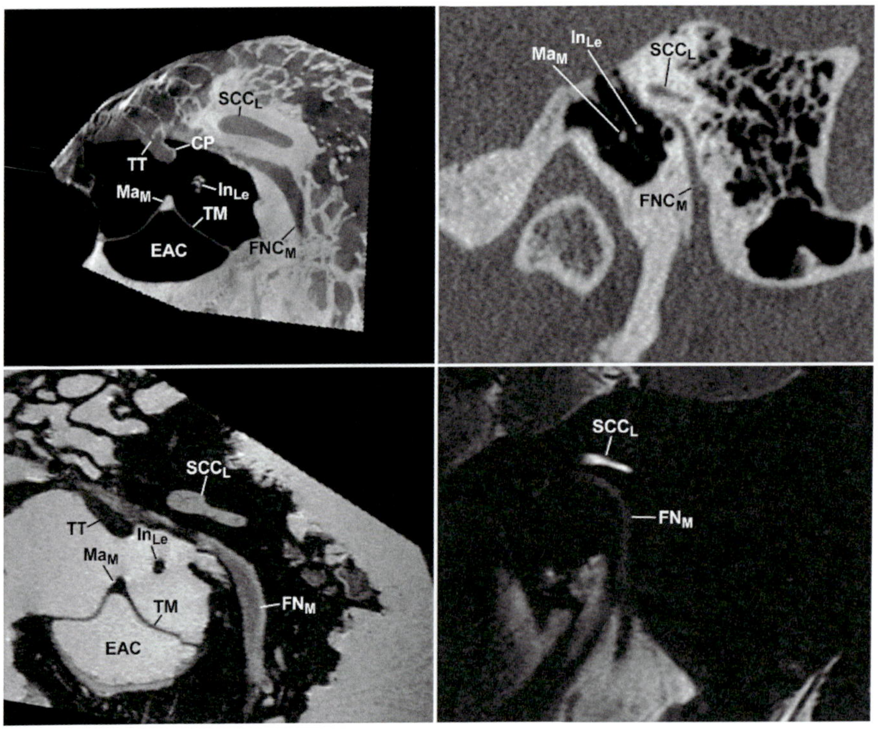
SCC_L
CP
TT
Ma_M
In_{Le}
TM
EAC
FNC_M
FN_M
Ma_M
In_{Le}
TT
SCC_L
FN_M

Fig. 71

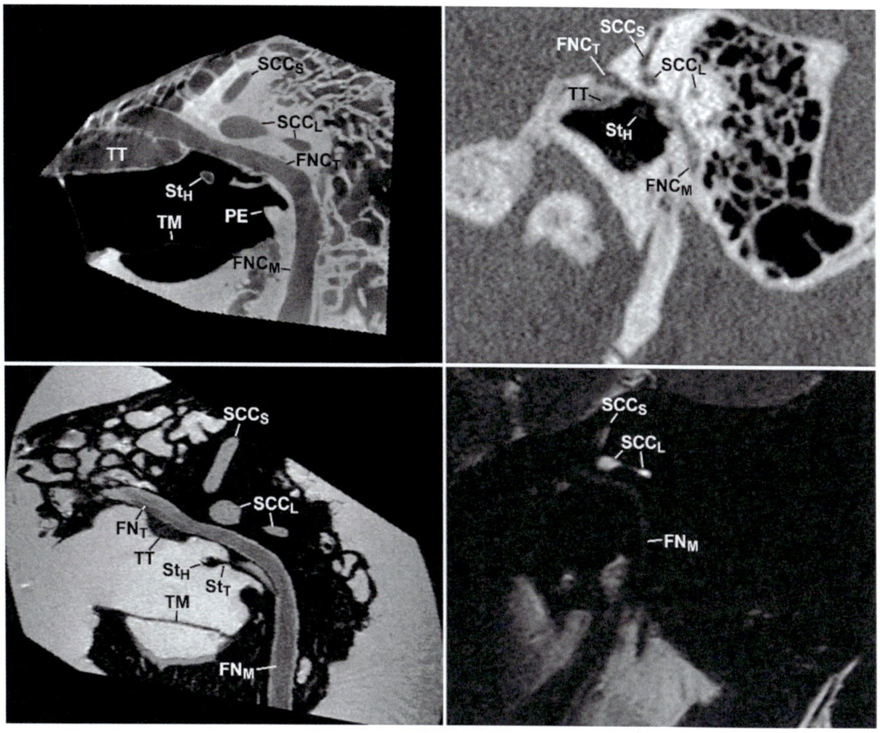
SCC_S
SCC_L
TT
FNC_T
St_H
TM
PE
FNC_M
SCC_S
FNC_T
SCC_L
TT
St_H
FNC_M
SCC_S
SCC_L
FN_T
TT
St_H
St_T
TM
FN_M
SCC_S
SCC_L
FN_M

Fig. 72

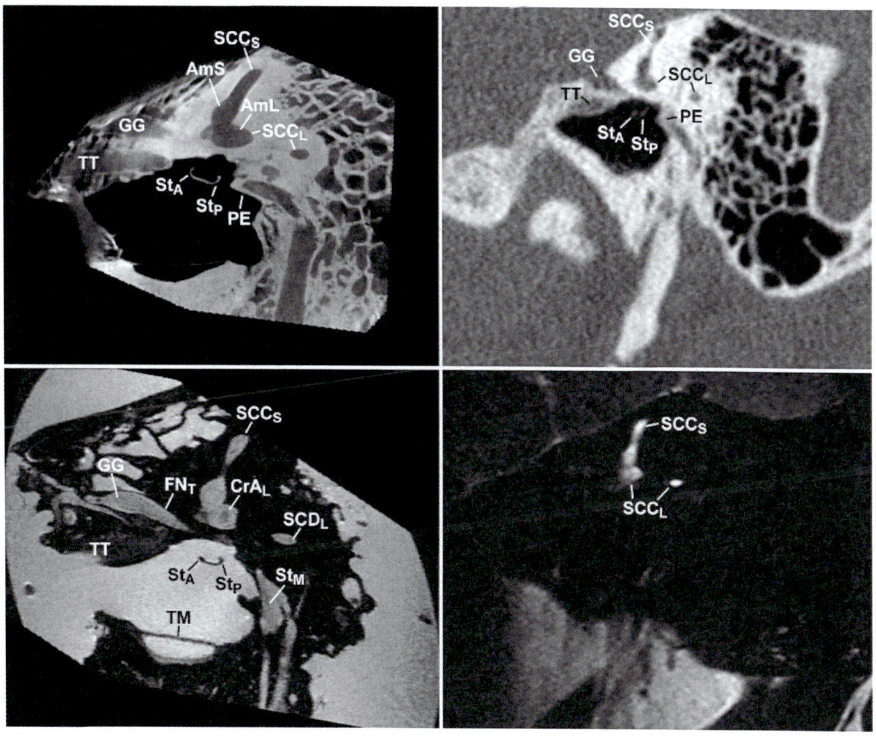
SCC_S
AmS
AmL
GG
SCC_L
TT
St_A
St_P
PE
SCC_S
GG
SCC_L
TT
PE
St_A
St_P
SCC_S
GG
FN_T
CrA_L
SCD_L
TT
St_A
St_P
St_M
TM
SCC_S
SCC_L

Fig. 73

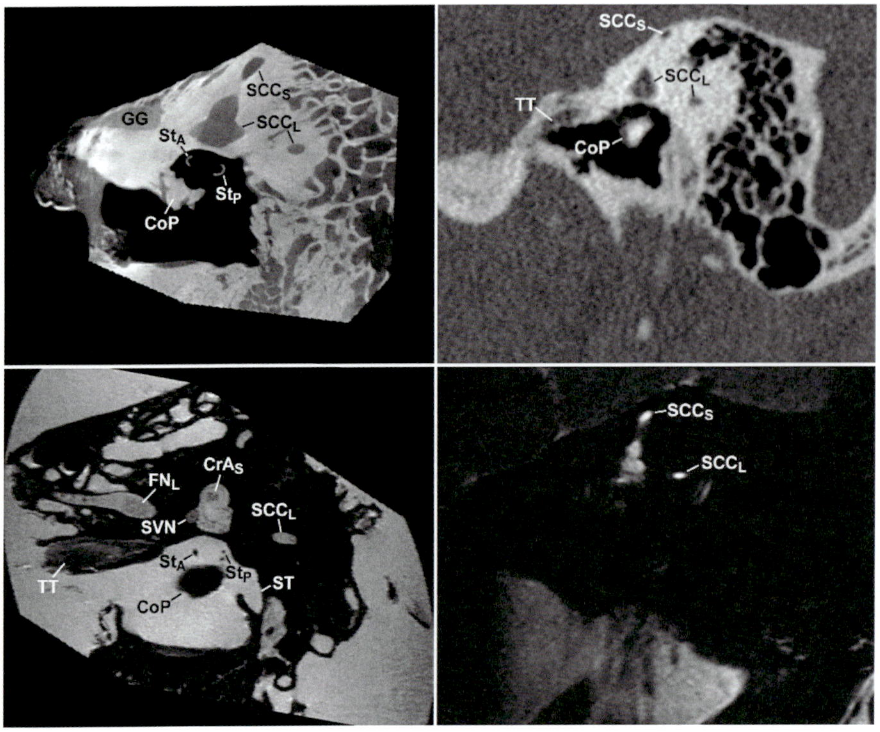
SCC$_S$
GG
St$_A$
SCC$_L$
St$_P$
CoP
SCC$_S$
SCC$_L$
TT
CoP
CrA$_S$
FN$_L$
SCC$_L$
SVN
St$_A$
St$_P$
ST
TT
CoP
SCC$_S$
SCC$_L$

Fig. 74

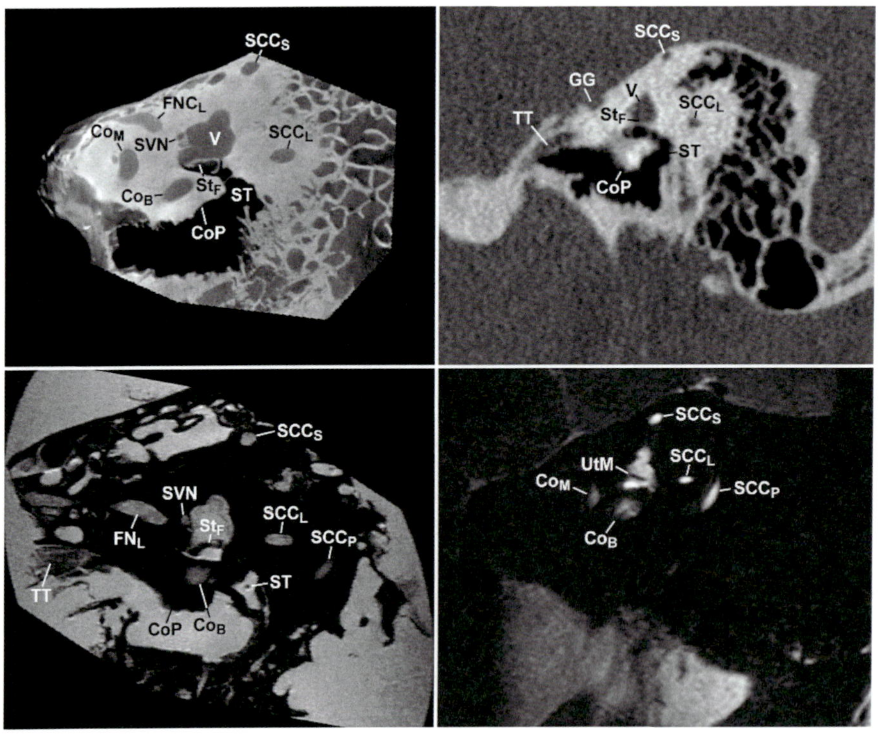
SCC$_S$
FNC$_L$
Co$_M$
SVN
V
SCC$_L$
St$_F$
ST
Co$_B$
CoP
SCC$_S$
GG
V
St$_F$
SCC$_L$
TT
ST
CoP
SCC$_S$
SVN
St$_F$
SCC$_L$
FN$_L$
SCC$_P$
TT
ST
CoP
Co$_B$
SCC$_S$
UtM
SCC$_L$
Co$_M$
SCC$_P$
Co$_B$

Fig. 75

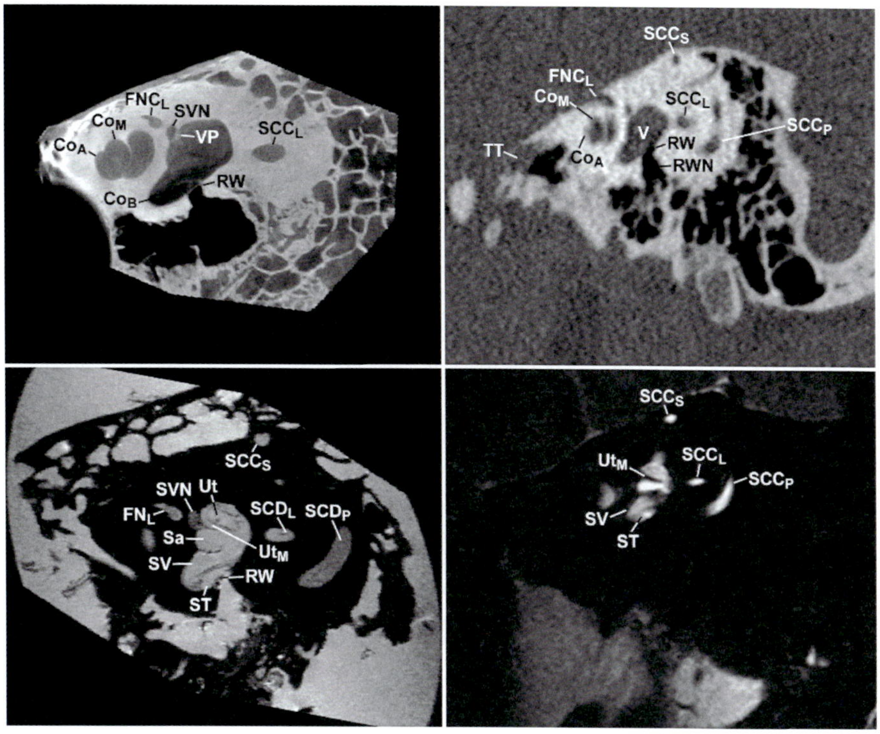

FNCL
CoM
SVN
CoA
VP
SCCL
RW
CoB
SCCS
FNCL
CoM
SCCL
V
RW
SCCP
TT
CoA
RWN
SCCS
SVN
Ut
FNL
SCDL
SCDP
Sa
UtM
SV
RW
ST
SCCS
UtM
SCCL
SCCP
SV
ST

Fig. 76

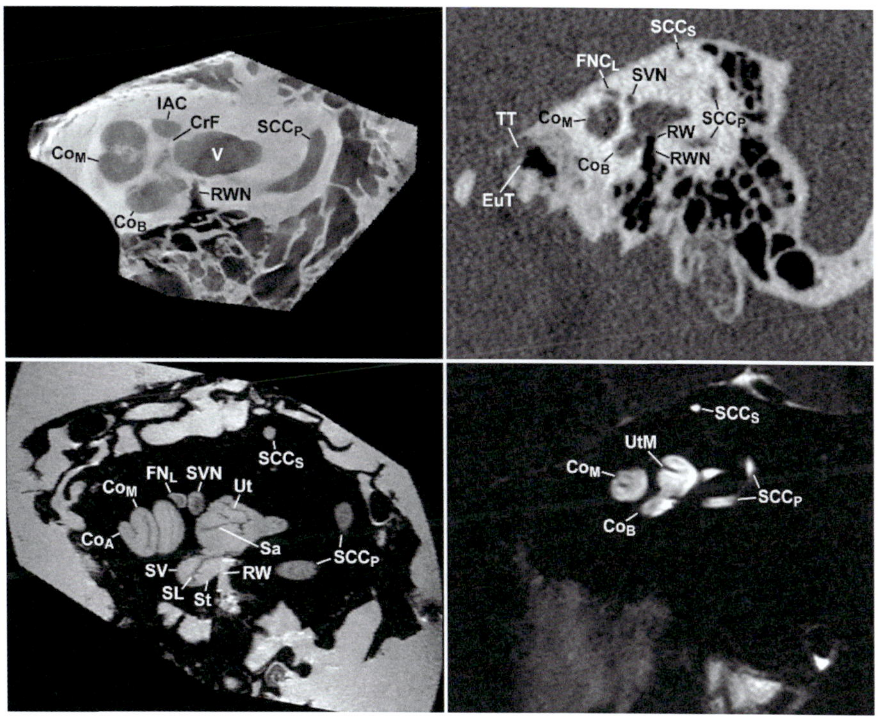

IAC
CrF
SCCP
CoM
V
RWN
CoB
SCCS
FNCL
SVN
TT
CoM
SCCP
RW
CoB
RWN
EuT
SCCS
FNL
SVN
CoM
Ut
CoA
Sa
SCCP
SV
RW
SL
St
SCCS
UtM
CoM
SCCP
CoB

Fig. 77

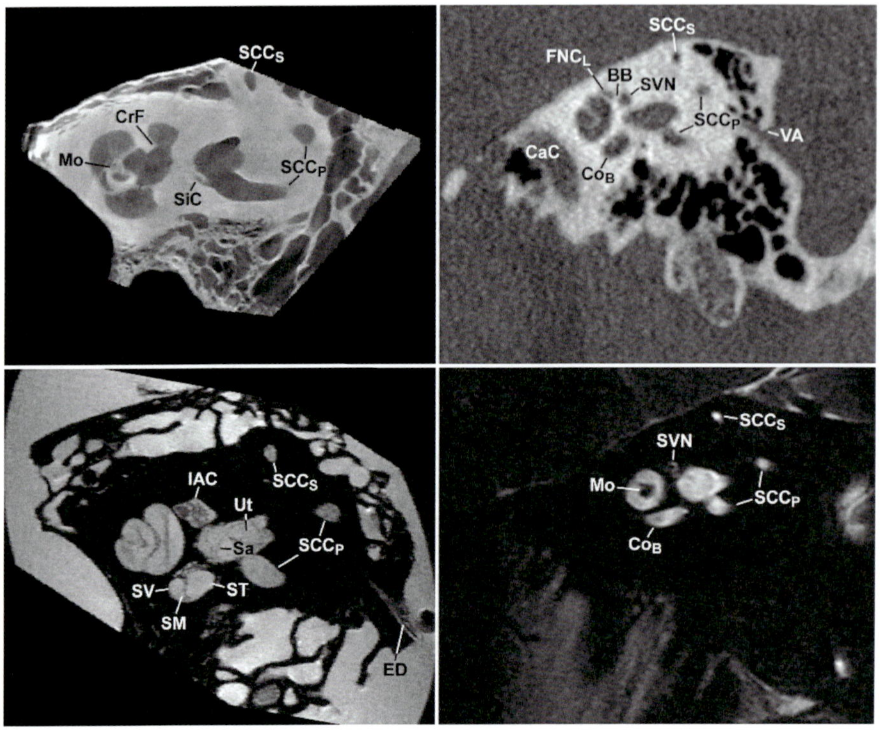
SCC_S
CrF
Mo
SiC
SCC_P
FNC$_L$
BB
SVN
VA
CaC
Co_B
IAC
Ut
Sa
SV
ST
SM
ED

Fig. 78

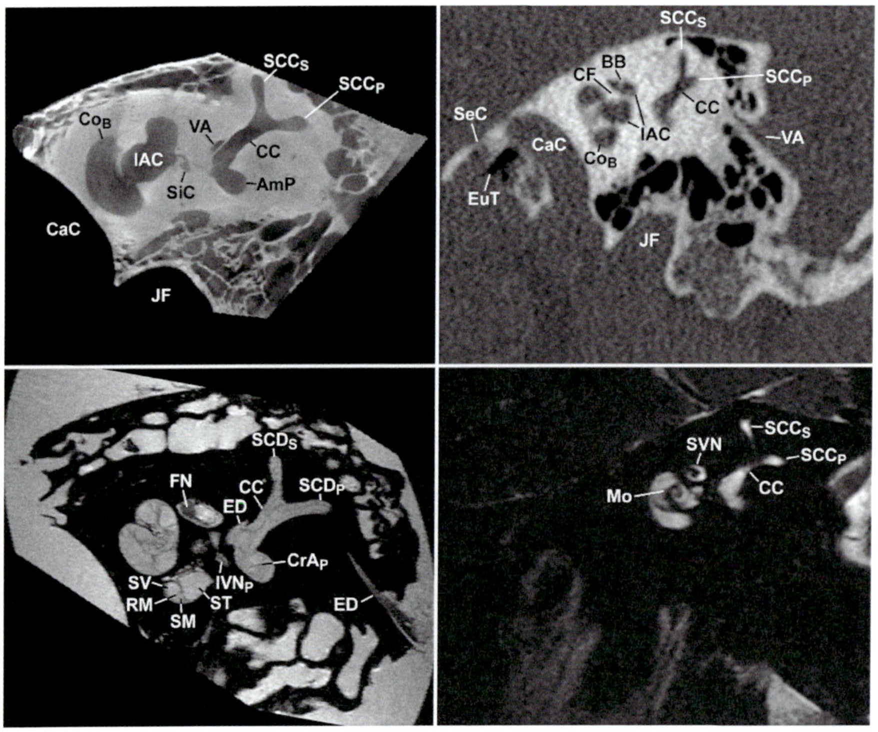
SCC_S
SCC_P
Co_B
VA
IAC
CC
SiC
AmP
CaC
JF
BB
CF
SeC
EuT
SCD_S
FN
ED
SCD_P
CrA$_P$
SV
RM
SM
IVN$_P$
ST
SVN
Mo

Fig. 79

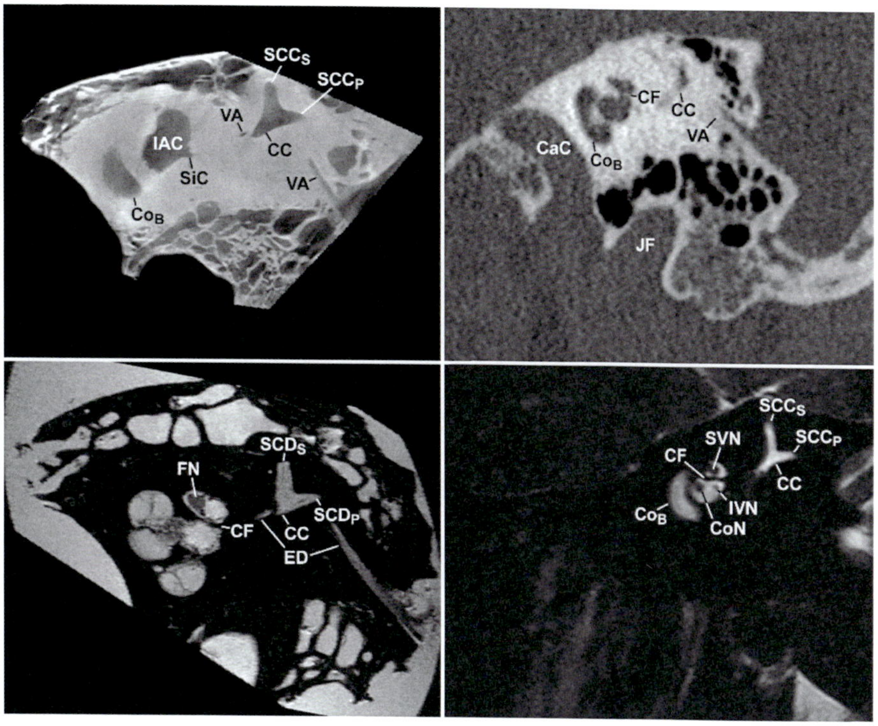
SCC_S
SCC_P
VA
IAC
CC
SiC
VA
Co_B
CF
CC
VA
CaC
Co_B
JF
SCD_S
FN
CF
CC
SCD_P
ED
SCC_S
SVN
SCC_P
CF
CC
Co_B
IVN
CoN

Fig. 80

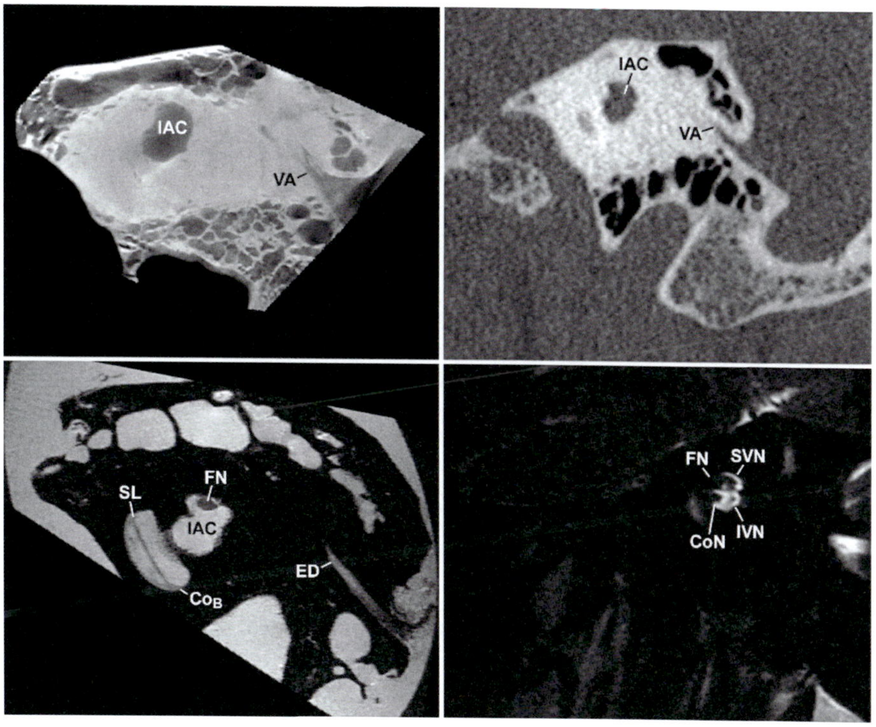
IAC
VA
IAC
VA
SL
FN
IAC
ED
Co_B
FN
SVN
CoN
IVN

Fig. 81

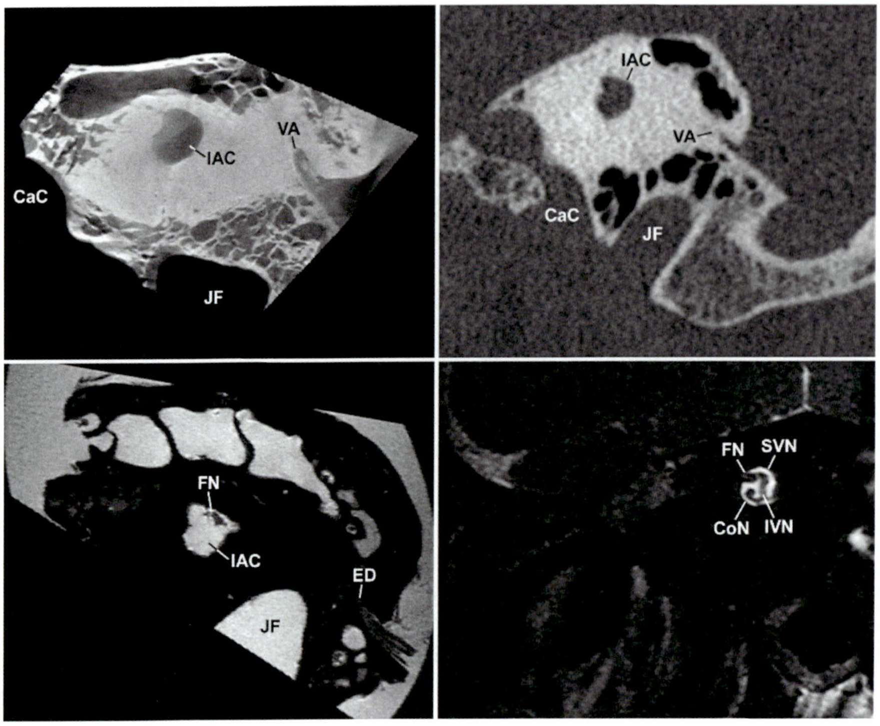

Fig. 82

References

1. Brunner S. Tomography in otoradiology. *Radiologe* 1969;9: 56–60
2. Buckingham RA, Valvassori GE. Tomographic anatomy of the temporal bone. *Otolaryngol Clin North Am* 1973;6: 337–362
3. Pimontel-Appel B, Ettore GC. Pöschl positioning and the radiology of ménière's disease. *J Belge Radiologie* 1980;63: 359–367

T-Bone Key	
AAA	Aditus Ad Antrum
Am	Ampulla (Superior, Lateral, Posterior)
At	Attic
BB	Bill's Bar
BM	Basilar Membrane
CaC	Carotid Canal
CC	Common Crus
ChT	Chorda Tympani
ChTC	Chorda Tympani Canal
Co	Cochlea (Basal, Middle, Apical)
CoAp	Cochlear Aperture
CoAq	Cochlear Aqueduct
CoN	Cochlear Nerve
CoP	Cochlear Promontory
CP	Cochleariform Process
CrA	Crista Ampullaris (Lateral, Posterior, Superior)
CF	Crista Falciformis
ED	Endolymphatic Duct
EuT	Eustachian Tube
FoI	Fossa Incudis
FNC	Facial Nerve Canal (Labyrinthine, Mastoid, Tympanic)
FN	Facial Nerve (Labyrinthine, Mastoid, Tympanic)
FR	Facial Recess
GG	Geniculate Ganglion
IAC	Internal Auditory Canal
In	Incus (Body, Long, Lenticular, Short)
IS	Interscalar Septum
IVN	Inferior vestibular nerve (Posterior, Saccular)
IVNC	Inferior Vestibular Nerve Canal
JF	Jugular Foramen
LMA	Suspensory Ligament, mallear anterior
LML	Suspensory Ligament, mallear lateral
LMS	Suspensory Ligament, mallear superior
LIP	Suspensory Ligament, incudal posterior
LSA	Suspensory Ligament, stapedial annular

T-Bone Key	
MA	Mastoid Antrum
Ma	Malleus (Anterior process, Head, Lateral process, Neck)
Mo	Modiolus
OW	Oval window
PE	Pyramidal Eminence
PS	Prussak's Space
RM	Reissner's Membrane
RW	Round Window
RWN	Round Window Niche
Sa	Saccule
SaM	Saccular Macula
Sc	Scutum
SCC	Semicircular Canal (Lateral, Posterior, Superior)
SCD	Semicircular Duct (Lateral, Posterior, Superior)
SeC	Semi Canal
SiC	Singular Canal
SiT	Sinus Tympani
SL	Spiral lamina
SM	Scala Media
ST	Scala Tympani
St	Stapes (Anterior crus, Footplate, Head, Neck, Posterior crus)
StM	Stapedial Muscle
StT	Stapedial Tendon
SV	Scala Vestibuli
SVN	Superior Vestibular Nerve
SVNC	Superior Vestibular Nerve Canal
TeT	Tegmen Tympani
TM	Tympanic Membrane
TT	Tensor Tympani
Ut	Utricle
UtM	Utricular Macula
V	Vestibule
VA	Vestibular Aqueduct
VP	Vestibular Pyramid

4 Advanced Imaging Applications

Since the advent of computed tomography (CT), the physical limitations of gantry angle and patient positioning have restricted the temporal bone imaging plane of section to standard axial and coronal projections. Most anatomical structures of the middle and inner ear are not optimally profiled in these planes. In the days of temporal bone polytomography complex oblique projections were often employed to show certain anatomical structures of the middle and inner ear to better effect. Recent advances in multidetector CT (MDCT) technology and high resolution 3D MR pulse sequences allow for the acquisition of volumetric data with isotropic voxel size permitting reconstructions in any plane of section. These postprocessing techniques have proven to be of benefit in the evaluation of both middle and inner ear pathological conditions [1–8].

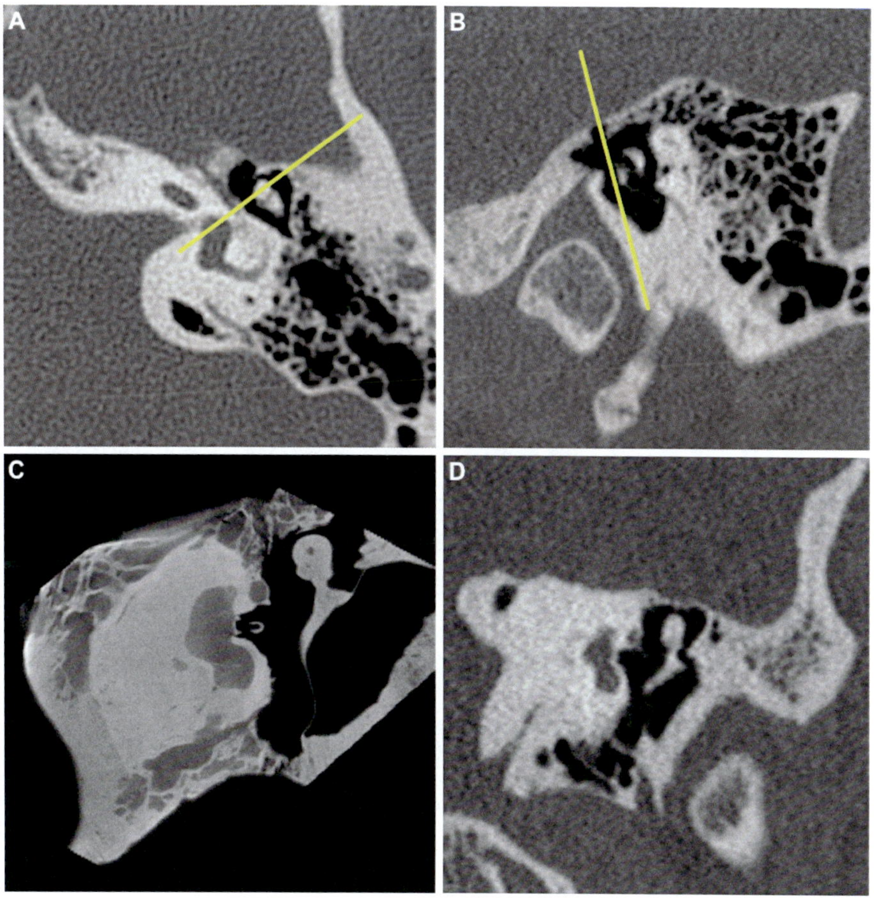

Fig. 1 Long axis oblique coronal reconstruction of the malleus. (**a**) Axial and (**b**) sagittal references images demonstrating multiplanar reconstruction (MPR) planes (yellow lines) required for the coronal long axis view of the malleus. (**c**) MPR of the malleus from the microCT dataset. (**d**) MPR of the malleus from the multidetector CT (MDCT) dataset

J. I. Lane, R. J. Witte, *The Temporal Bone*, DOI: 10.1007/978-3-642-02210-4_4,

In this chapter, we demonstrate some of the optimal imaging planes that can be used to display normal anatomy as well as pathological conditions involving the middle and inner ear. Most of the multiplanar reconstructions (MPRs) employed in this chapter are slight modifications of the imaging planes displayed in the Chap. 3 (axial, coronal, Pöschl, Stenvers).

Because of the limitations of MR in distinguishing air from adjacent cortical bone, MDCT is the modality of choice in the imaging of the middle ear structures. MR is helpful as an adjunct in characterizing soft tissue masses occupying the middle ear space and for assessing intracranial extension of disease.

Long axis MPRs and maximum intensity projections (MIPs) of the ossicles can be useful in excluding subtle fixation or erosion in the setting of chronic inflammatory disease, fracture/dislocation in the setting of temporal bone trauma, and congenital ossicular anomalies (Figs. 1–9). Pöschl plane reconstructions of the ossicles provide an ideal depiction of both the incomallear and incostapedial articulations (Figs. 10–12). MPRs in the plane of the long and short axis of the

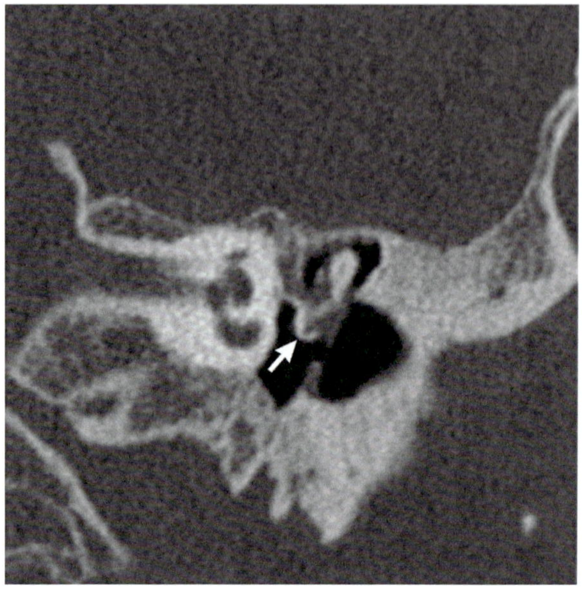

Fig. 2 Clinical application: long axis oblique coronal reconstruction of the malleus. Extensive tympanosclerosis demonstrated by calcified chronic inflammatory tissue (*arrow*) causes fixation and medial displacement of the manubrium of the malleus in this patient with conductive hearing loss

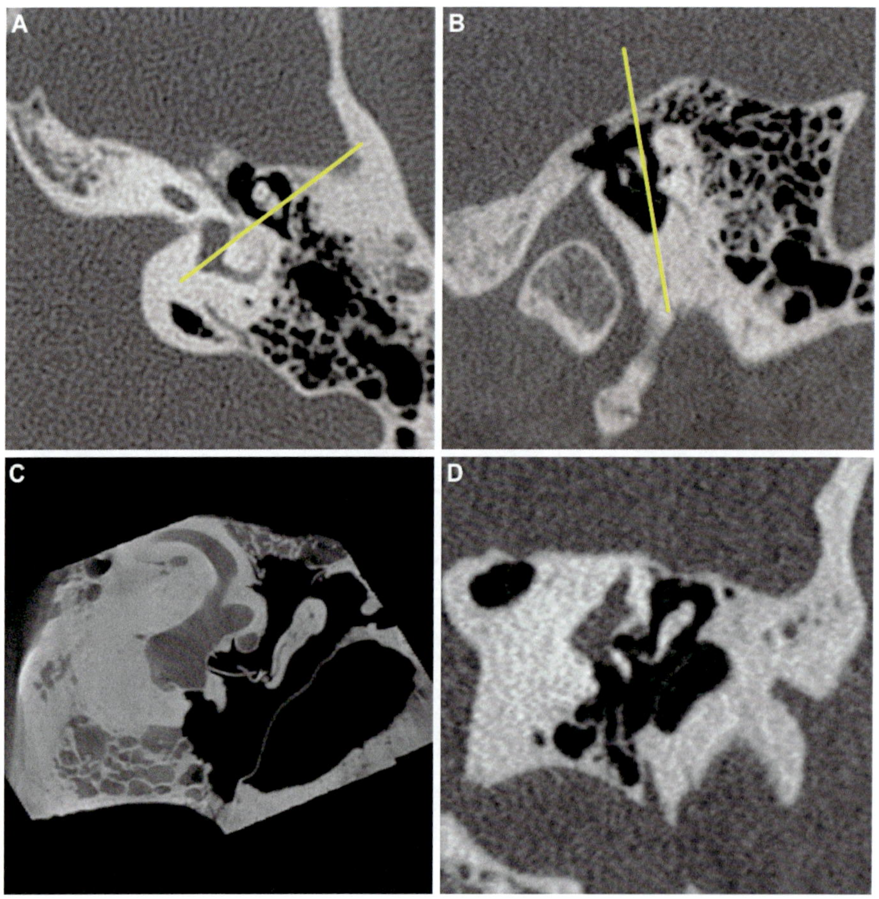

Fig. 3 Long axis oblique coronal reconstruction of the incus. (**a**) Axial and (**b**) sagittal references images demonstrating MPR planes (yellow lines) required for the coronal long axis view of the incus. (**c**) MPR of the incus from the microCT dataset. (**d**) MPR of the incus from the MDCT dataset

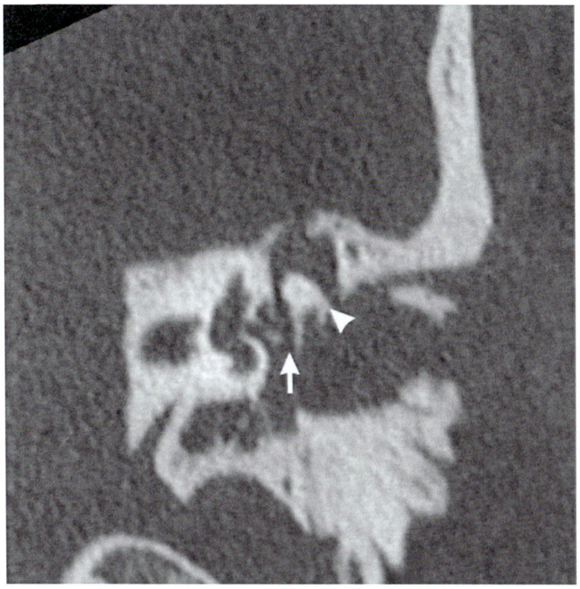

Fig. 4 Clinical application: long axis oblique coronal reconstruction of the incus. Incostapedial disarticulation (*arrow*) with rotational dislocation of the incus. Note the short process is rotated laterally from its normal posterior orientation (*arrowhead*) in this patient with acute longitudinal fracture of the left temporal bone

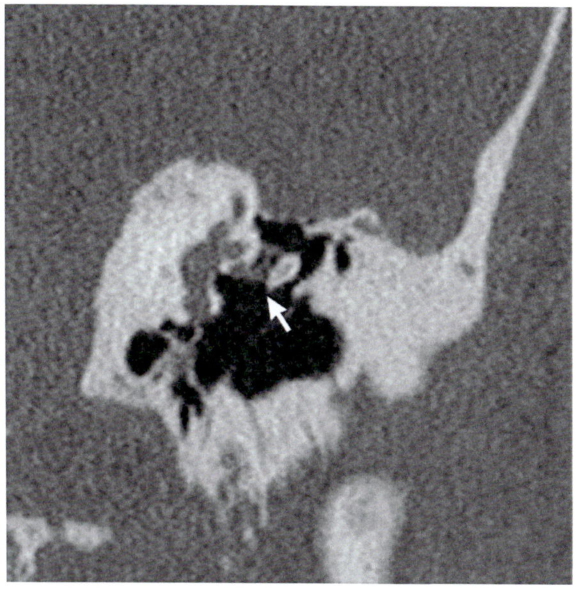

Fig. 5 Clinical application: long axis oblique coronal reconstruction of the incus. Eroded long process of the incus (*arrow*) with incostapedial disarticulation in this patient with conductive hearing loss

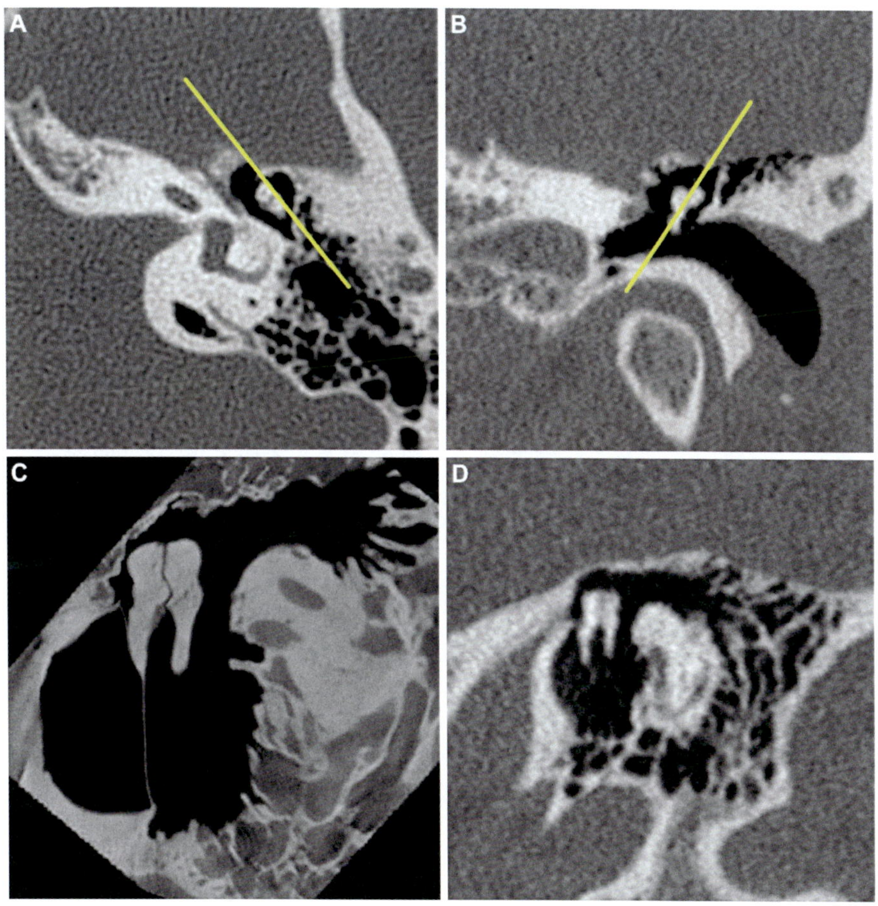

Fig. 6 Long axis oblique sagittal reconstruction of the malleus and incus (molar tooth view). (**a**) Axial and (**b**) coronal reference images demonstrating MPR planes (yellow lines) required to view the sagittal long axis of the malleus and incus. (**c**) MPR of the malleus and incus from the microCT dataset. (**d**) MPR of the malleus and incus from the MDCT dataset. (**e**) Maximum intensity projection (MIP) of the malleus and incus from the microCT dataset (2-mm slab). (**f**) MIP of the malleus and incus from the MDCT dataset (2-mm slab). Note the normal relationship of the malleus anterior to the incus with the mallear head articulating with the articular facet of the incus

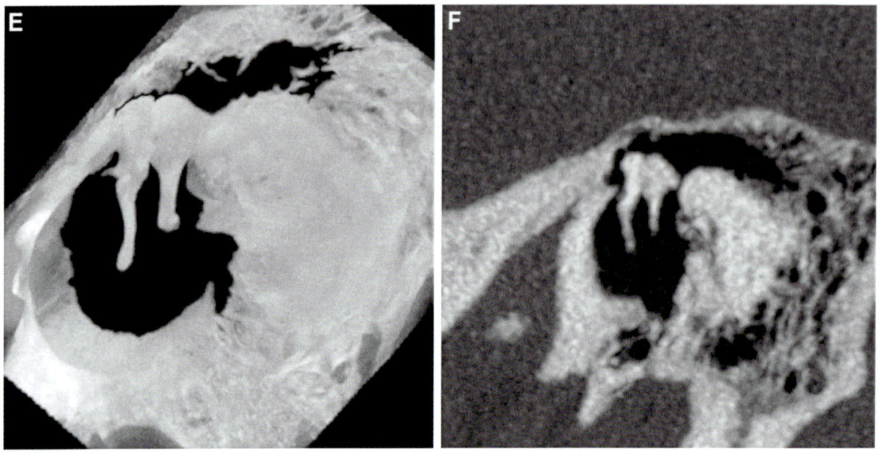

Fig. 6 (continued)

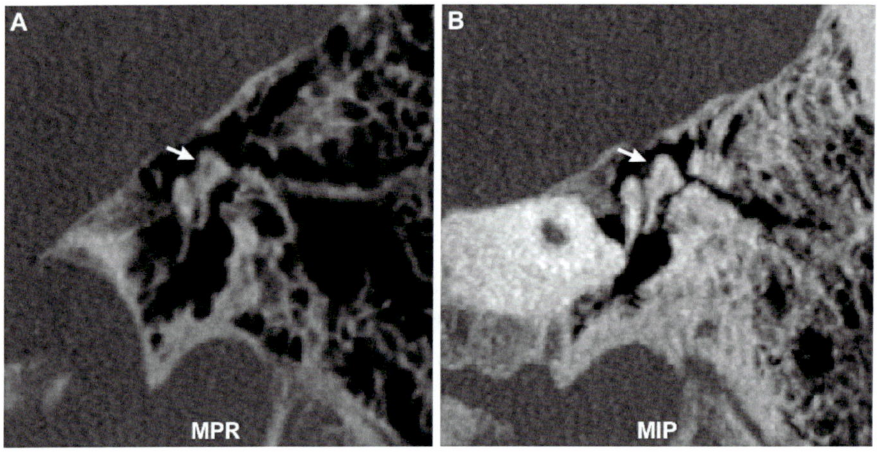

Fig. 7 Clinical application: long axis oblique sagittal reconstruction of the malleus and incus (molar tooth view). Remote traumatic disarticulation of the malleus and incus. (**a**) MPR and (**b**) MIP (2-mm slab) of the disarticulated malleus and incus. Note the "empty" articular facet of the incus (*arrow*) with the inferiorly displaced malleus relative to the incus

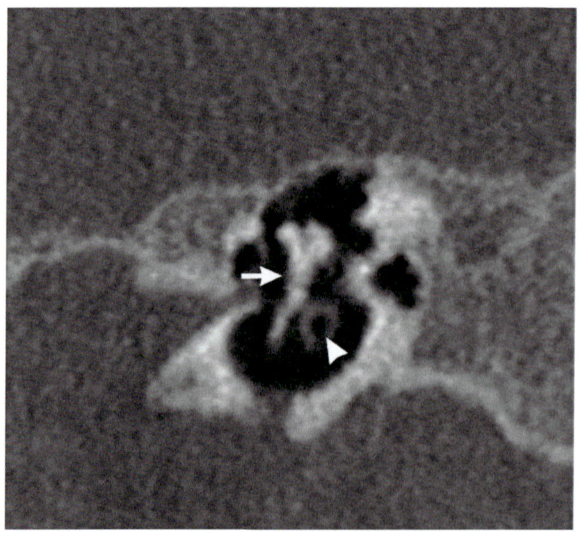

Fig. 8 Clinical application: long axis oblique sagittal reconstruction of the malleus and incus (molar tooth view). Fused malleus and incus (*arrow*) in this patient with microtia and hypoplastic middle ear. Incidental note made of a tympanostomy tube (*arrowhead*)

stapes are helpful in displaying subtle otospongiotic (otosclerotic) lesions causing stapes fixation (Figs. 13–16).

Inner ear disease can be evaluated with MDCT or high resolution MR. These modalities can often be complementary. MR is the modality of choice for the evaluation of disease processes involving the internal auditory canal, providing direct visualization of the 7th and 8th nerves. Both modalities can be used in assessing normal labyrinthine anatomy (Figs. 17–35) and in the detection of labyrinthine anomalies associated with congenital deafness or early sensorineural hearing loss (Figs. 22, 26, and 28). MPRs of volumetric data can be useful in the assessment of localized defects of the bony labyrinth, such as erosion or dehiscence of the semicircular canals (Figs. 30, 32, and 34). MDCT is useful in the detection of postinflammatory or posttraumatic calcification of the labryinthine structures (labyrinthitis ossificans) and MPRs can aid in localizing and assessing the extent of this calcification (Figs. 18, 22, 35).

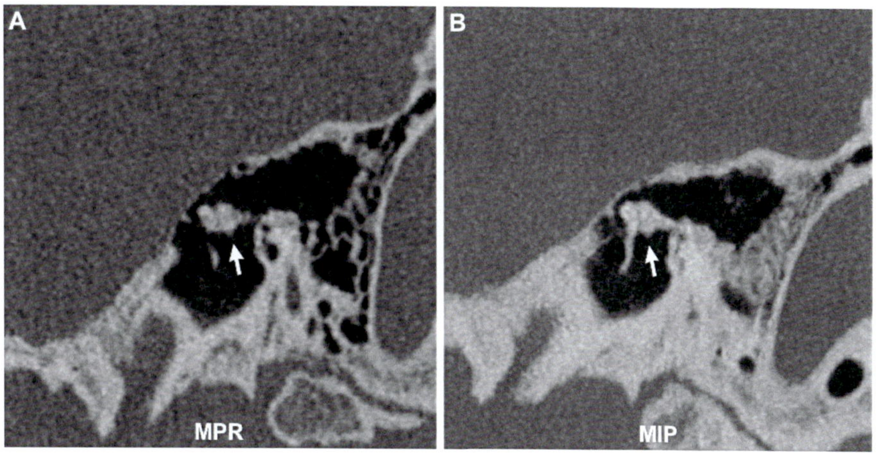

Fig. 9 Clinical application: long axis oblique sagittal reconstruction of the malleus and incus (molar tooth view). Eroded long process of the incus. (**a**) MPR and (**b**) MIP (2-mm slab) demonstrating amputated long process (*arrow*) posterior to an intact manubrium of the malleus (same patient as in Fig. 5)

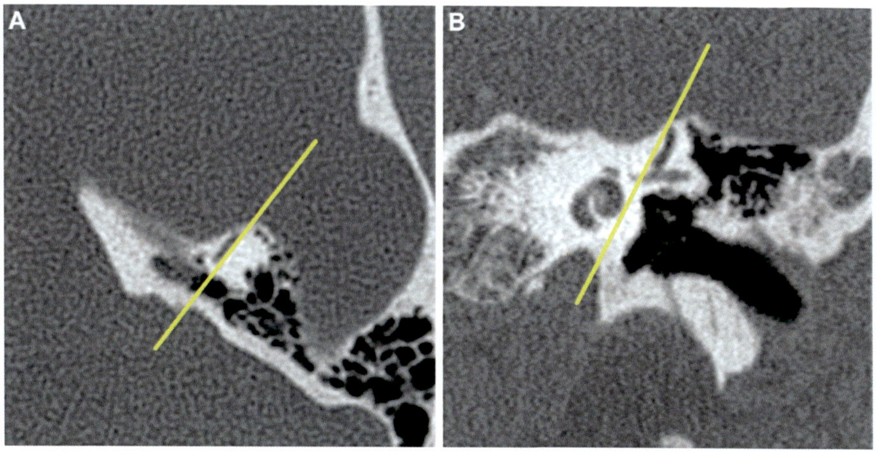

Fig. 10 Pöschl plane reconstruction of the malleus and incus. (**a**) Axial and (**b**) coronal references images demonstrating MPR in the plane of the superior semicircular canal (yellow lines) required for this view of the malleus and incus. (**c**) MPR of the malleus and incus from the microCT dataset. (**d**) MPR of the malleus and incus from the MDCT dataset. (**e**) MIP of the malleus and incus from the microCT dataset (2-mm slab). (**f**) MIP of the malleus and incus from the MDCT dataset (2-mm slab). Note the normal relationship of the manubrium of the malleus lateral to the long process of the incus in this projection

Fig. 10 (continued)

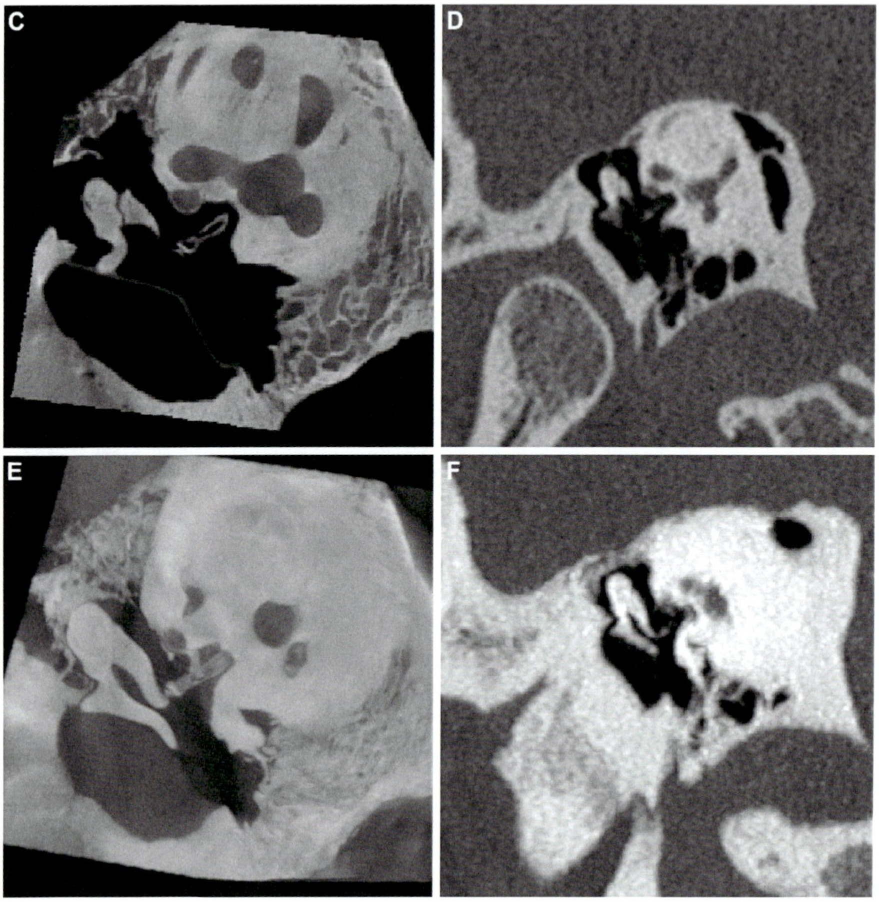

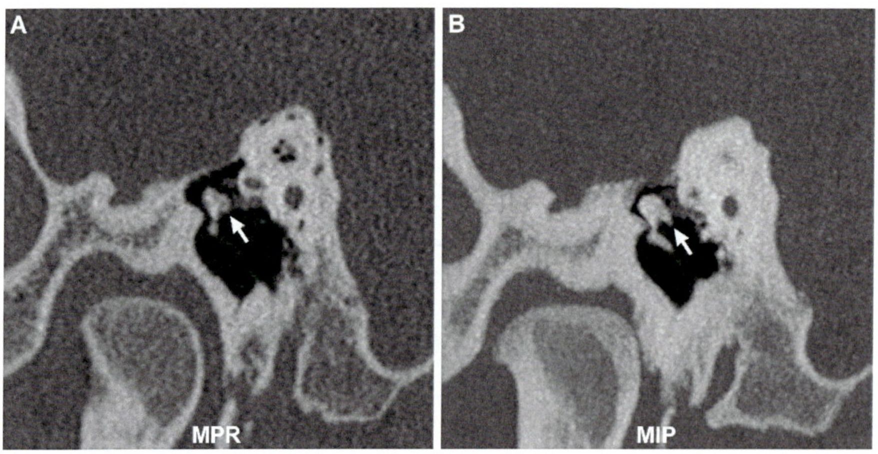

Fig. 11 Clinical application: Pöschl plane reconstruction of the malleus and incus. Eroded long process of the incus. (**a**) MPR and (**b**) MIP demonstrating the amputated long process (*arrow*) medial to an intact manubrium of the malleus (same patient as in Fig. 5)

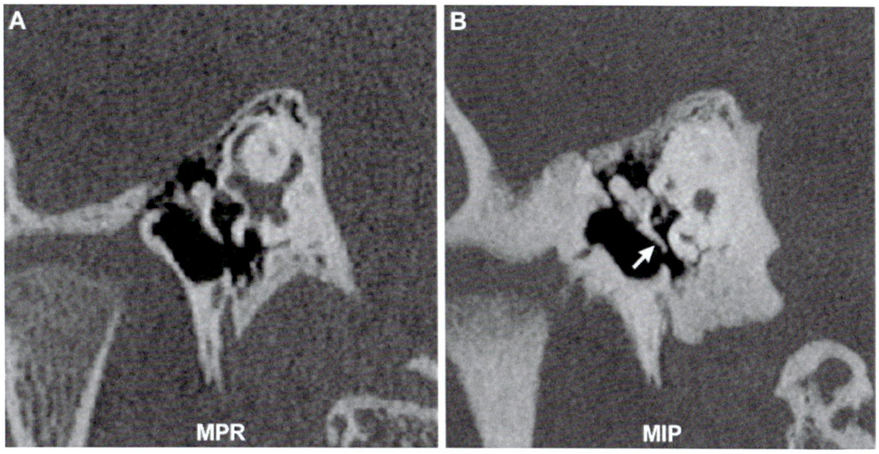

Fig. 12 Clinical application: Pöschl plane reconstruction of the malleus and incus. Remote traumatic disarticulation of the malleus and incus. (**a**) MPR and (**b**) MIP (2-mm slab) demonstrating disarticulation of the malleus and incus. The malleus and incus are no longer seen together in the same plane on the MPR. MIP demonstrates that the head of the malleus is inferiorly displaced relative to the body of the incus and the manubrium of the malleus (*arrow*) is displaced medial to the long process of the incus (same patient as in Fig. 7)

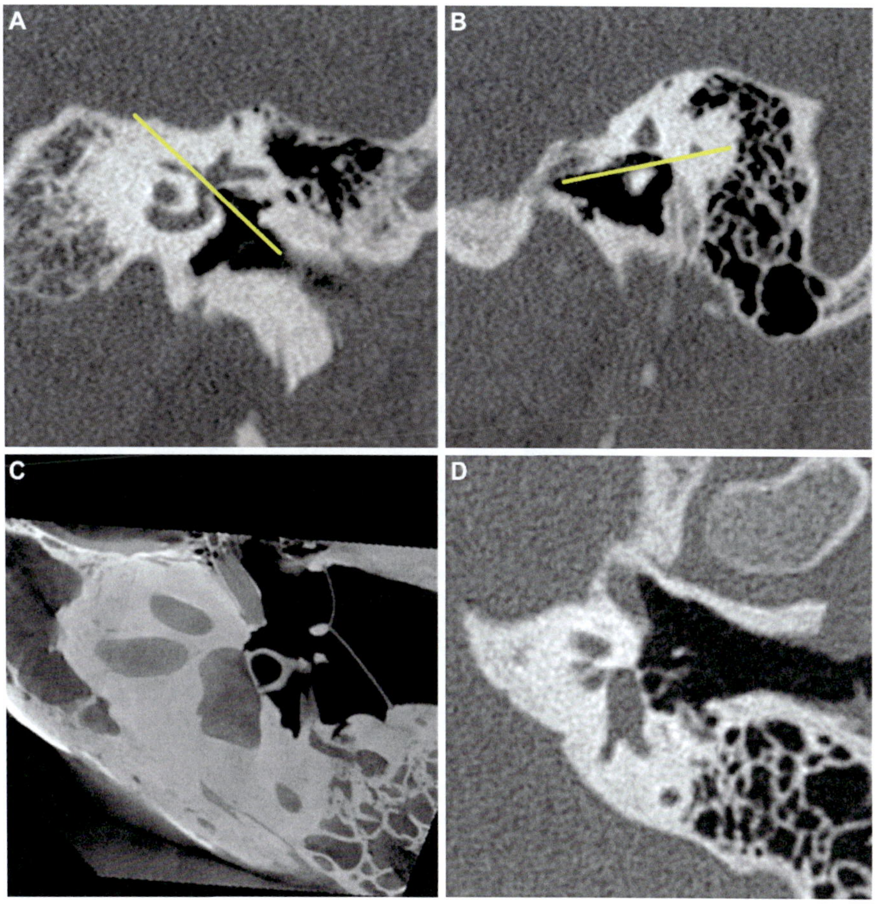

Fig. 13 Long axis oblique axial reconstruction of the stapes. (**a**) Coronal and (**b**) sagittal reference images demonstrating MPR planes (yellow lines) required for the long axis oblique axial view of the stapes. (**c**) MPR of the incus from the microCT dataset. (**d**) MPR of the stapes from the MDCT dataset

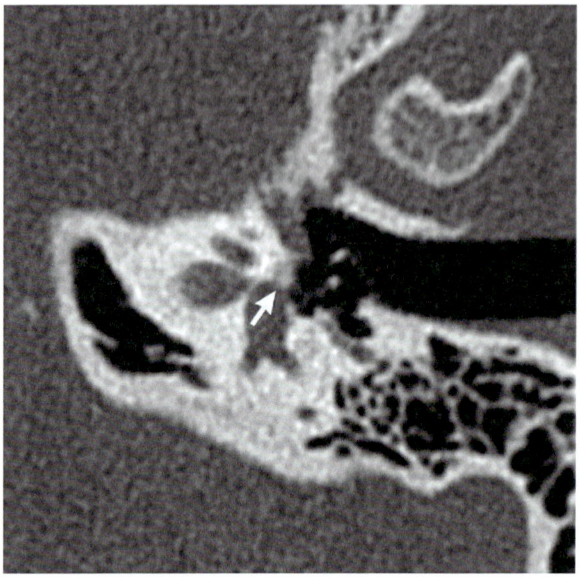

Fig. 14 Clinical application: long axis oblique axial reconstruction of the stapes. Fixation of the footplate and anterior crus of the stapes secondary to fenesteral otospongiosis. Note the stapes seen in the long axis with demineralized, otospongiotic bone arising from the region of the fissula antefenestrum and encasing the anterior edge of the footplate and anterior crus (*arrow*)

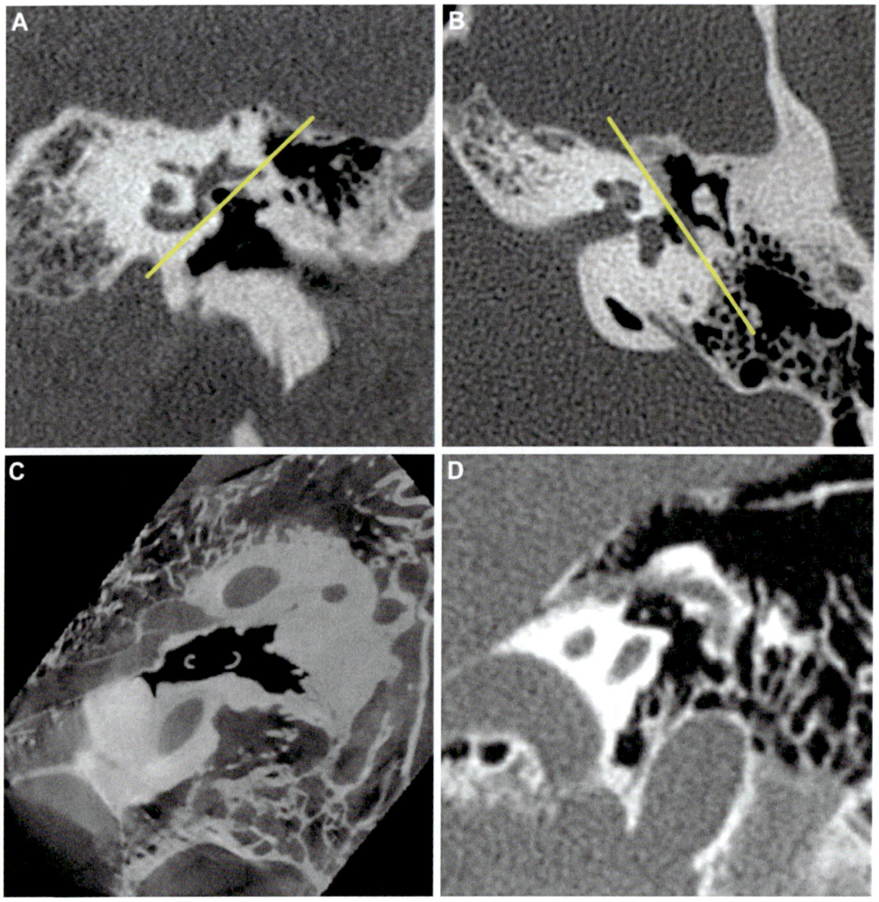

Fig. 15 Short axis oblique sagittal reconstruction of the stapes. (**a**) Coronal and (**b**) axial reference images demonstrating MPR planes (yellow lines) required for the short axis oblique sagittal view of the stapes. (**c**) MPR of the stapes from the microCT dataset. (**d**) MPR of the stapes from the MDCT dataset. Note the anterior and posterior crura in cross-section within the oval window niche

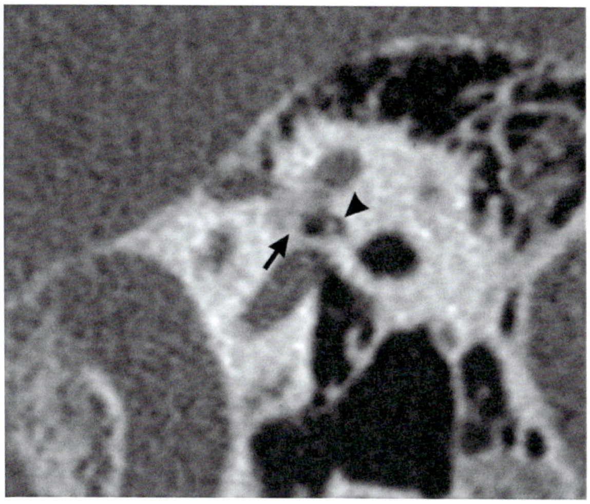

Fig. 16 Clinical application: short axis oblique sagittal reconstruction of the stapes. Fixation of the footplate and anterior crus of the stapes secondary to fenesteral otospongiosis. Note the stapes seen in the short axis with demineralized, otospongiotic bone arising from the region of the fissula antefenestrum and encasing the anterior crus (*arrow*). Note that the posterior crus is not involved (*arrowhead*)

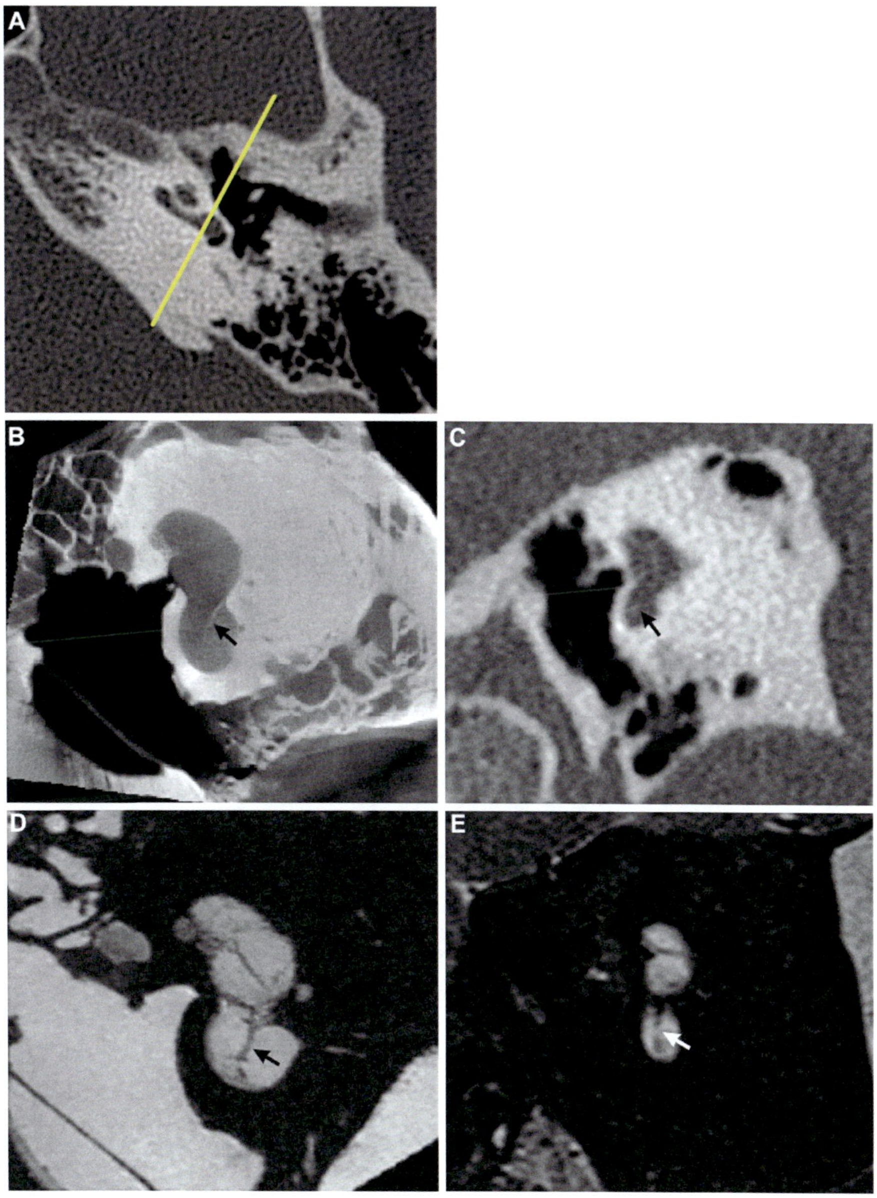

Fig. 17 Oblique sagittal reconstruction through the basal turn of the cochlea. (**a**) Axial reference images demonstrating the MPR plane (yellow line) required for the oblique sagittal view through the basal turn of the cochlea. The angle of reconstruction is identical to that of the Pöschl plane. MPR through the basal turn from (**b**) the microCT and (**c**) the MDCT datasets. MPR through the basal turn from (**d**) the microMR and (**e**) 3T MR datasets. Note the position of the spiral lamina (*arrow*), partitioning the basal turn into the anterior scala vestibuli and posterior scala tympani

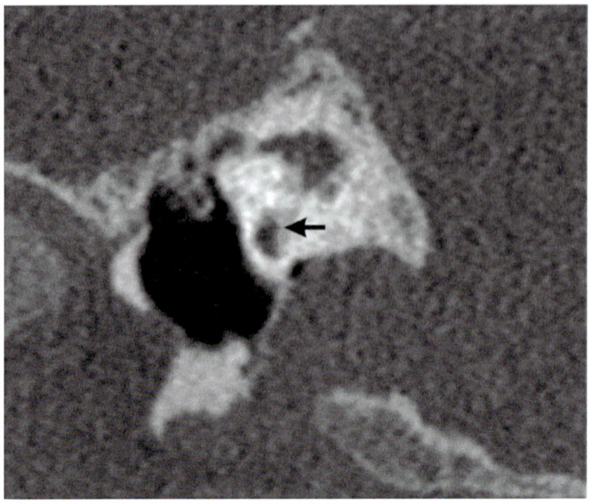

Fig. 18 Clinical application: oblique sagittal reconstruction through the basal turn of the cochlea. Pre-operative MDCT for a cochlear implant demonstrates ossification of the scala tympani (*arrow*) within the posterior portion of the basal turn secondary to remote labyrinthitis (labyrinthitis ossificans). Recognition of the ossification being limited to the scala tympani of the basal turn may convince the surgeon to place the electrode array more anteriorly into the patent scala vestibuli

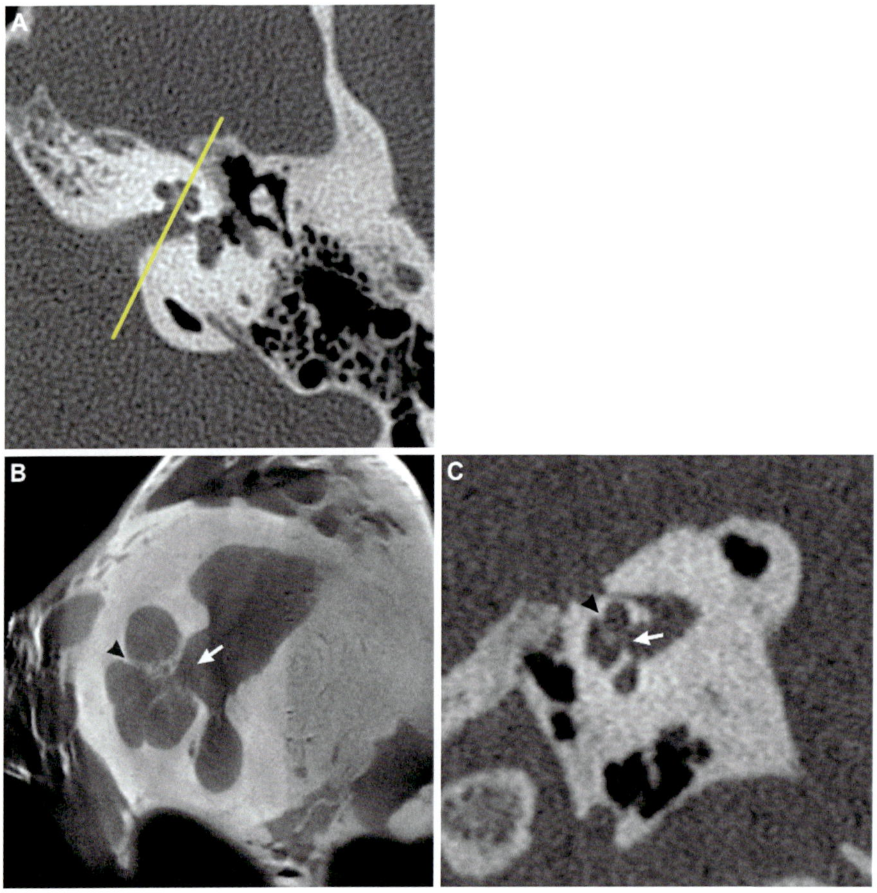

Fig. 19 Oblique sagittal reconstruction through the modiolus of the cochlea. (**a**) Axial reference images demonstrating the MPR plane (yellow line) required for the oblique sagittal view through the modiolus of the cochlea. The angle of reconstruction is identical to that of the Pöschl plane. MPR through the modiolus from (**b**) the microCT and (**c**) the MDCT datasets. MPR through the modiolus from (**d**) the microMR and (**e**) the 3T MR datasets. Note the relationship of the cochlear nerve hiatus to the base of the modiolus (*arrow*) and the notched indentation to the superior contour of the cochlea at the site of the interscalar septum, separating the basal from the middle turn (*arrowhead*)

Fig. 19 (continued)

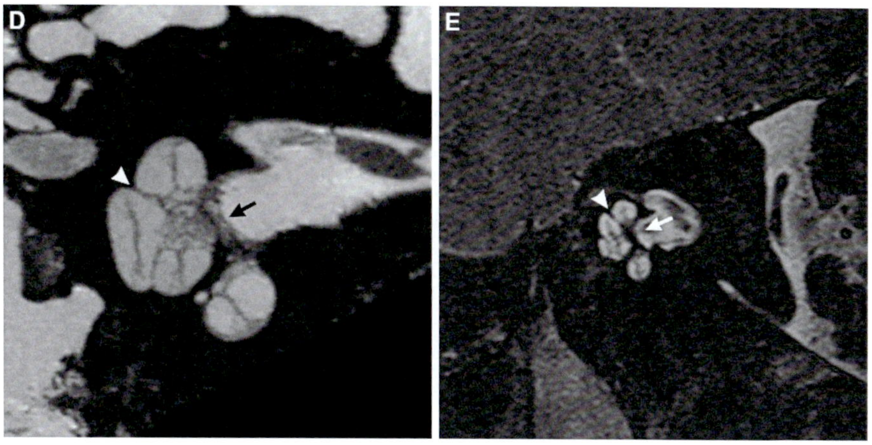

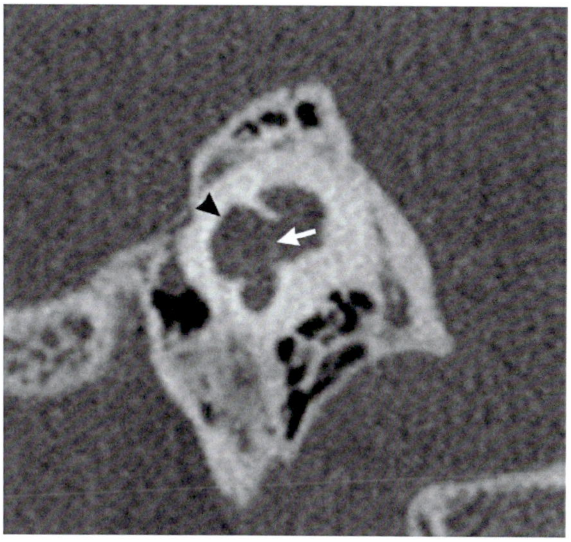

Fig. 20 Clinical application: oblique sagittal reconstruction through the modiolus of the cochlea. MDCT reconstruction in a child with Mondini malformation and profound sensorineural hearing loss demonstrates widened cochlear nerve hiatus and deficient modiolus (*arrow*). Note the partition anomaly of the cochlea demonstrated by loss of the normal notched indentation of the superior contour of the cochlea (*arrowhead*). These findings are typical of Mondini malformation

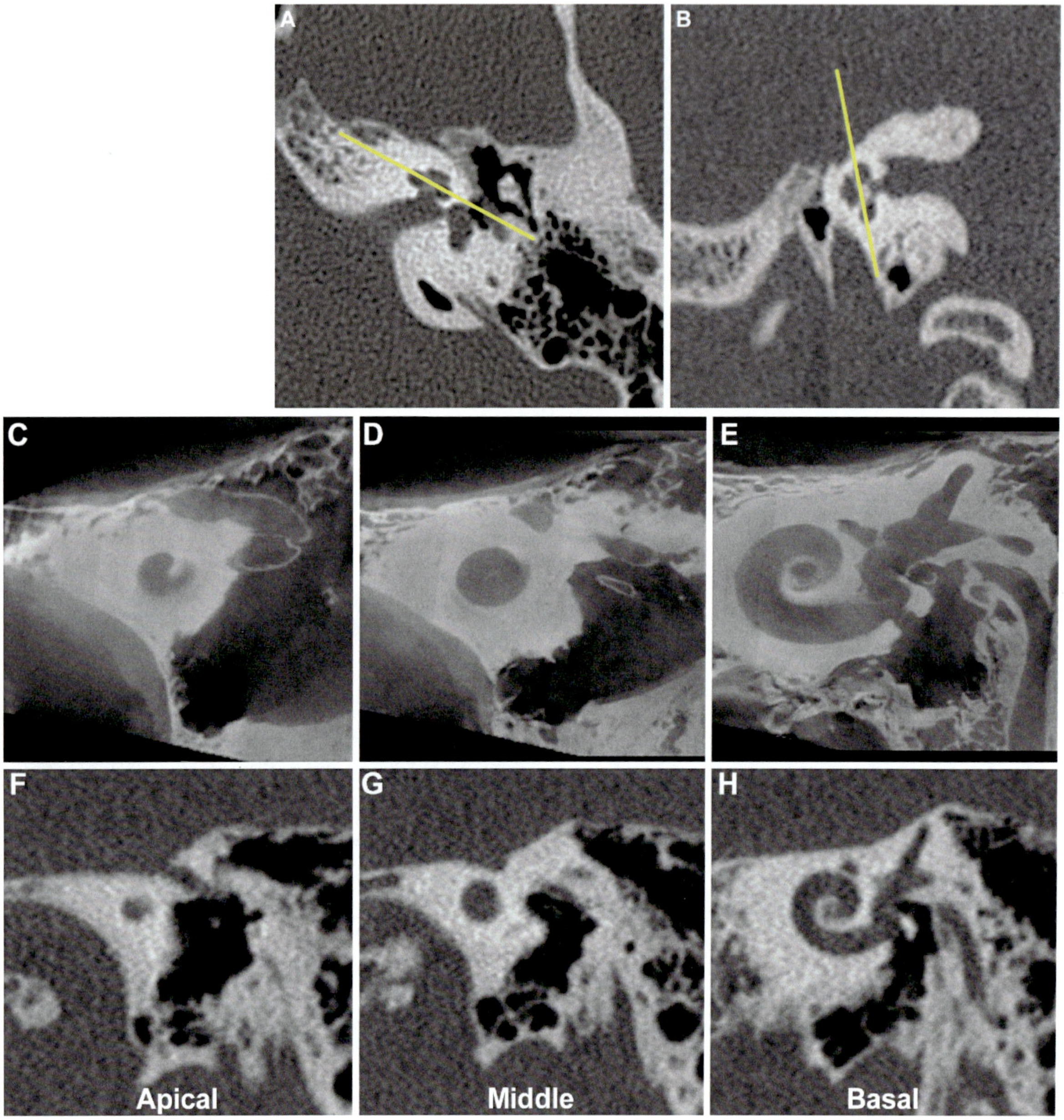

Fig. 21 Oblique coronal reconstruction through the turns of the cochlea. (**a**) Axial and (**b**) sagittal reference images demonstrating the MPR planes (yellow lines) required for the oblique coronal views through the turns of the cochlea. The angles of reconstruction are slight modifications of the Stenvers plane. MPRs of the cochlear turns from (**c**–**e**) the microCT and (**f**–**h**) the MDCT datasets. MPRs of (**i**–**k**) the cochlear turns from the microMR and (**l**–**n**) the 3T MR datasets

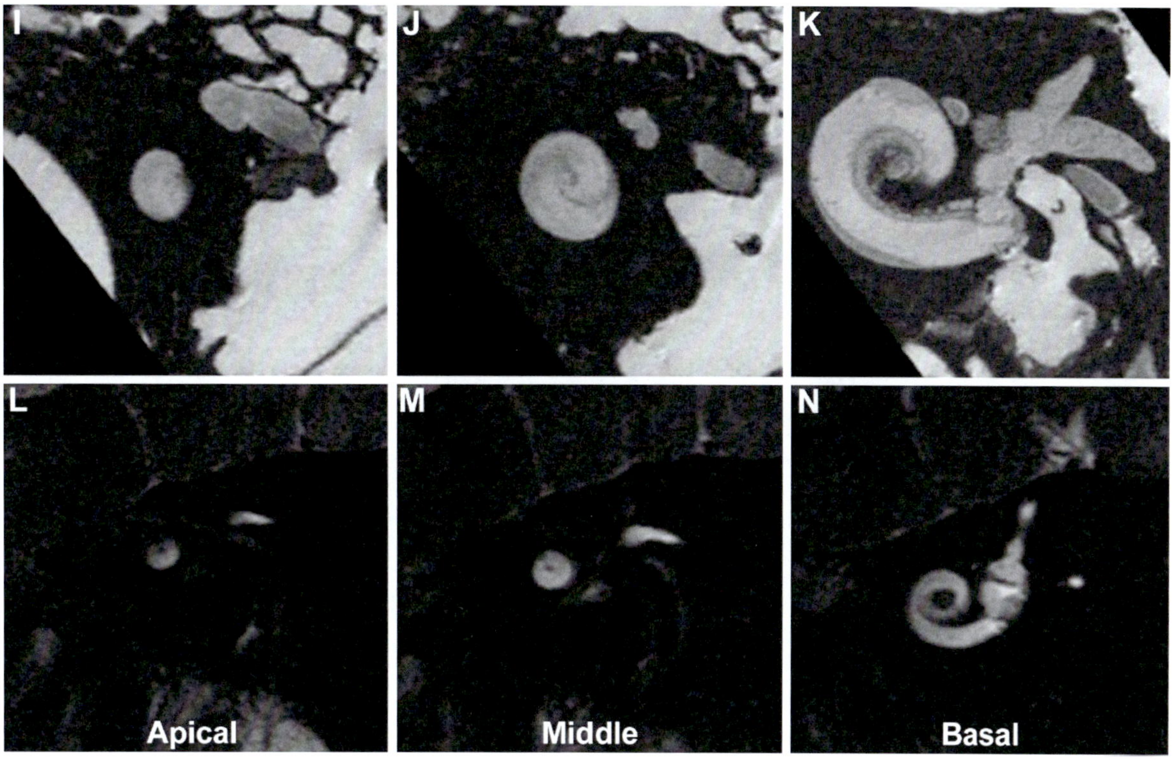

Fig. 21 (continued)

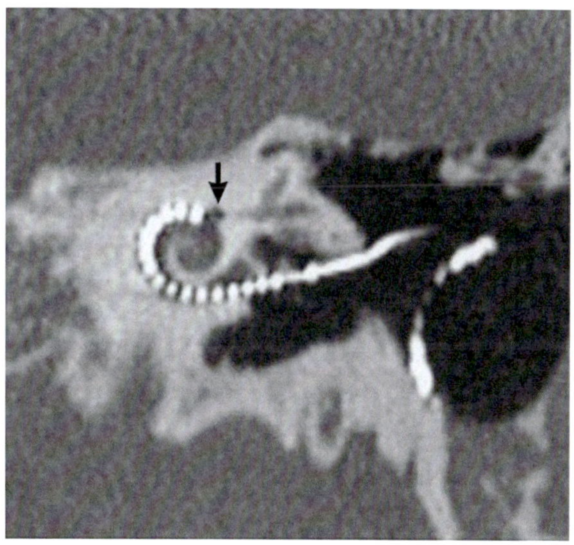

Fig. 22 Clinical application: oblique coronal reconstruction of the basal turn of the cochlea. This view of the cochlea is ideal for measuring the depth of insertion of the electrode array in patients with a cochlear implant. This patient was experiencing facial stimulation after implant insertion. The distal electrode is noted adjacent to the labyrinthine segment of the facial nerve (*arrow*). After MDCT had demonstrated this relationship, the distal electrode was selectively turned off and the symptoms resolved

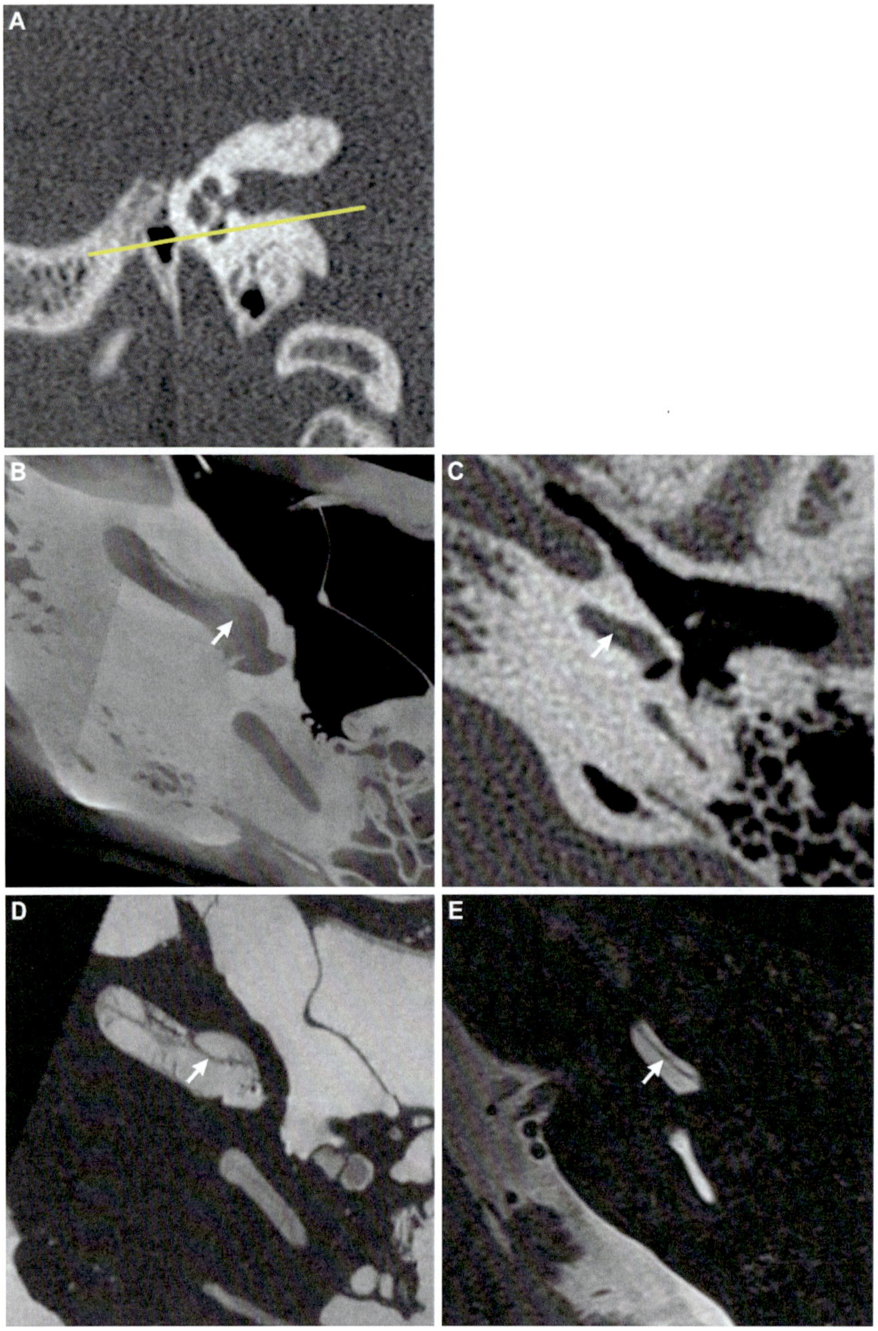

Fig. 23 Oblique axial reconstruction through the basal turn of the cochlea. (**a**) Sagittal reference image demonstrating the MPR plane (yellow line) required for the oblique axial view of the basal turn of the cochlea. MPR through the basal turn from (**b**) the microCT and (**c**) the MDCT datasets. MPR through (**d**) the basal turn from the microMR and (**e**) 3T MR datasets. Note the position of the spiral lamina (*arrow*) partitioning the cochlea into the anterior scala vestibuli and the posterior scala tympani

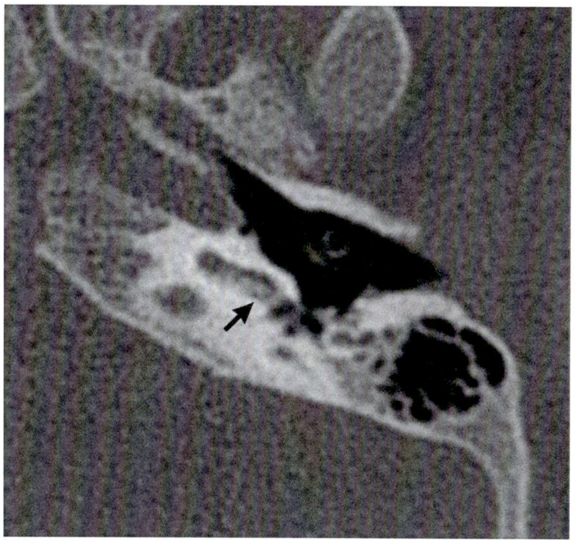

Fig. 24 Clinical application: oblique axial reconstruction through the basal turn of the cochlea. Pre-operative MDCT for a cochlear implant demonstrates ossification of the scala tympani (arrow) within the posterior portion of the basal turn, secondary to remote labyrinthitis (labyrinthitis ossificans). Recognition of the ossification being limited to the scala tympani of the basal turn may convince the surgeon to place the electrode array more anteriorly into the patent scala vestibuli

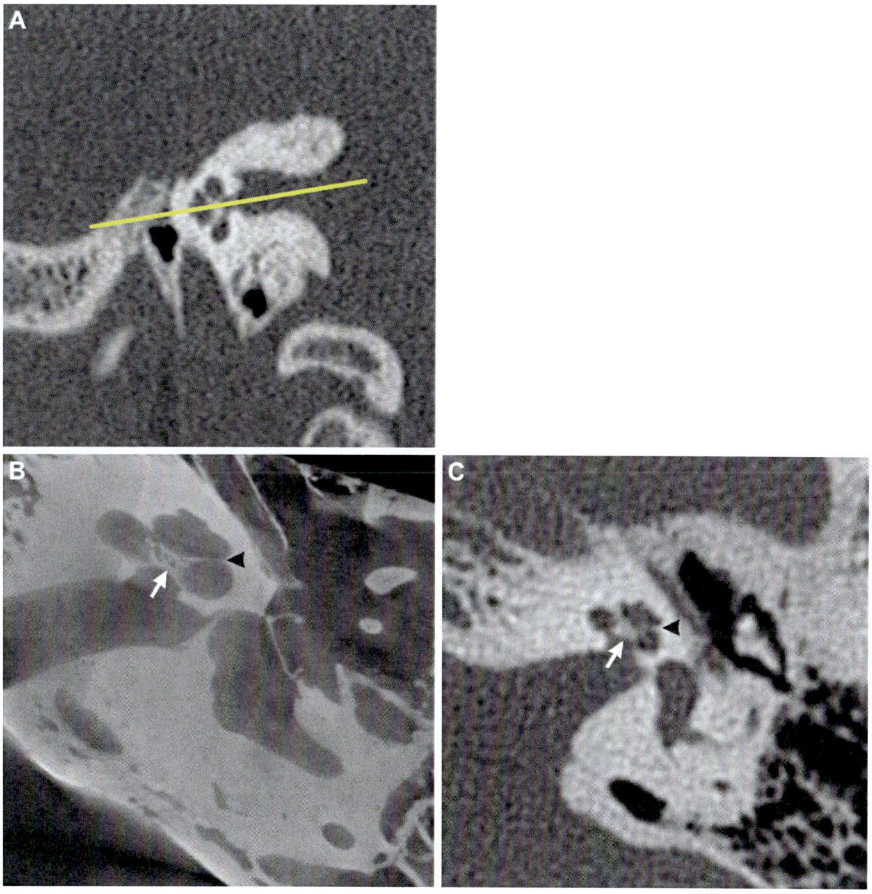

Fig. 25 Oblique axial reconstruction through the modiolus of the cochlea. (**a**) Sagittal reference images demonstrating the MPR plane (yellow line) required for the oblique sagittal view through the modiolus of the cochlea. MPR through the modiolus from (**b**) the microCT and (**c**) the MDCT datasets. MPR through the modiolus from (**d**) the microMR and (**e**) 3T MR datasets. Note the relationship of the cochlear nerve hiatus to the base of the modiolus (*arrow*) and the notched indentation to the lateral contour of the cochlea at the site of the interscalar septum, separating the basal from the middle turn (*arrowhead*)

Fig. 25 (continued)

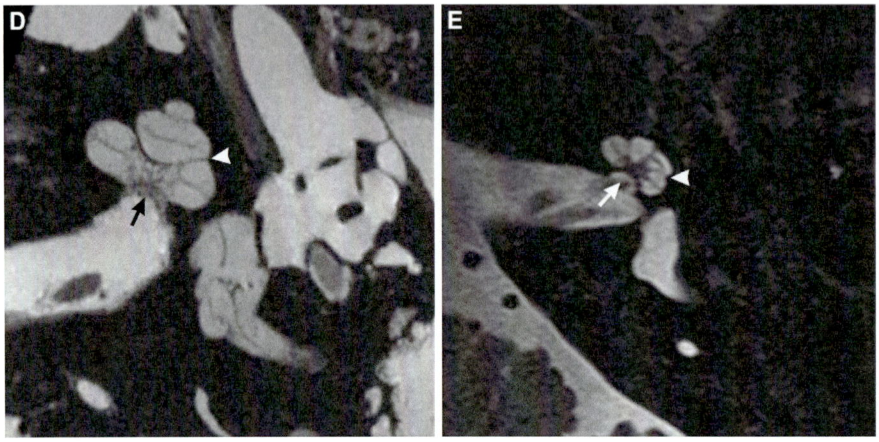

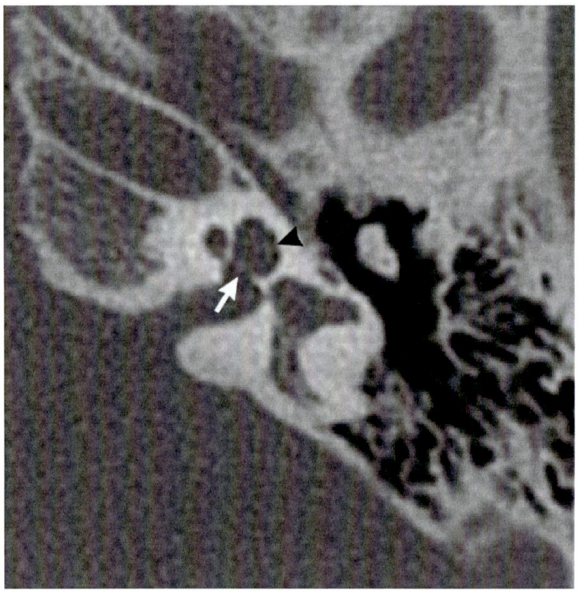

Fig. 26 Clinical application: oblique axial reconstruction through the modiolus of the cochlea. MDCT reconstruction in a child with Mondini malformation and profound sensorineural hearing loss demonstrates deficient modiolus (*arrow*). Note the partition anomaly of the cochlea demonstrated by loss of the normal notched indentation of the lateral contour of the cochlea (*arrowhead*). These findings are typical of Mondini malformation

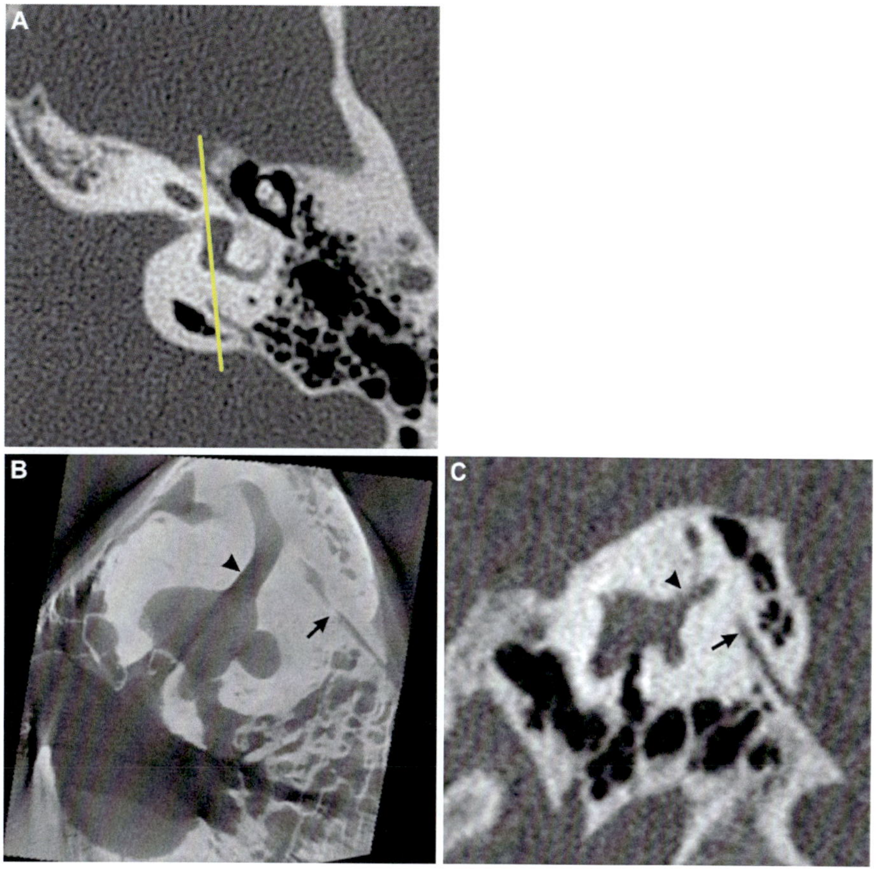

Fig. 27 Oblique sagittal reconstruction of the vestibular aqueduct. (**a**) Axial reference image demonstrating the reconstruction (MPR) plane (yellow line) required for the oblique sagittal view of the vestibular aqueduct. (**b**) MPR of the vestibular aqueduct from the microCT dataset. (**c**) MPR of the vestibular aqueduct from the MDCT dataset. Note that the vestibular aqueduct (*arrow*) courses anterosuperiorly from the posterior surface of the petrous temporal bone toward the common crus (*arrowhead*). The vestibular aqueduct opens along the medial wall of the vestibule just anterior and inferior to the opening of the common crus (see Chapter 2, Figs. 15–21). The midportion of the vestibular aqueduct should be no larger in caliber than the adjacent semicircular canals

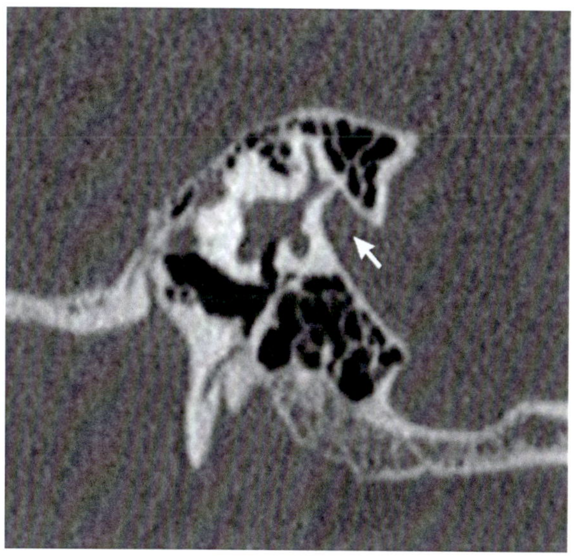

Fig. 28 Clinical application: oblique sagittal reconstruction of the vestibular aqueduct. MDCT reconstruction of a dilated vestibular aqueduct (arrow) in a patient presenting with progressive sensorineural hearing loss

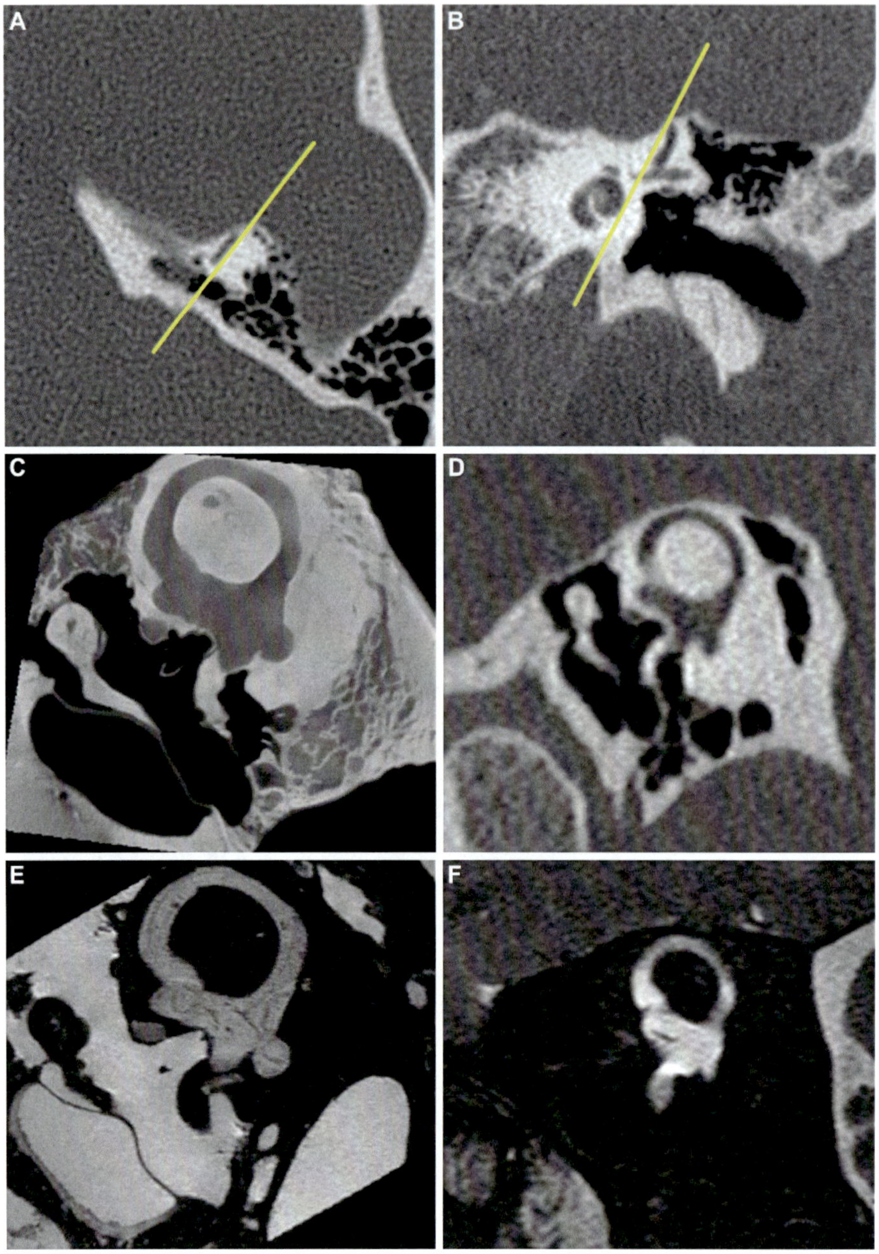

Fig. 29 Oblique sagittal reconstruction of the superior semicircular canal. (**a**) Axial and (**b**) coronal reference images demonstrating the MPR planes (yellow lines) required for the oblique sagittal view of the superior semicircular canal. The angle of reconstruction is identical to that of the Pöschl plane. MPR of the superior semicircular canal from (**c**) the microCT and (**d**) the MDCT datasets. MPR of the superior semicircular canal from (**e**) the microMR and (**f**) the 3T MR datasets

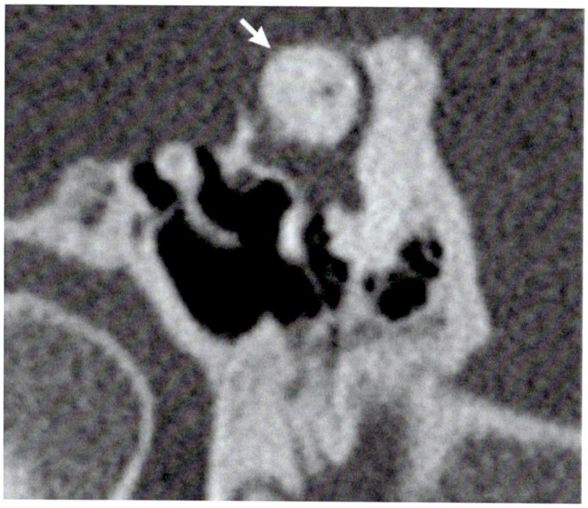

Fig. 30 Clinical application: oblique sagittal reconstruction of the superior semicircular canal. MDCT reconstruction in a patient presenting with vertigo precipitated by loud sounds (Tullio's phenomenon). Note dehiscence of the roof of the canal (arrow) allowing the defect to act as a "third window." In these patients the fluid wave generated at the oval window (first window) can decompress at the site of the dehiscence rather than at the round window (second window). This abnormal route of fluid wave propagation stimulates the vestibular apparatus, resulting in vertigo

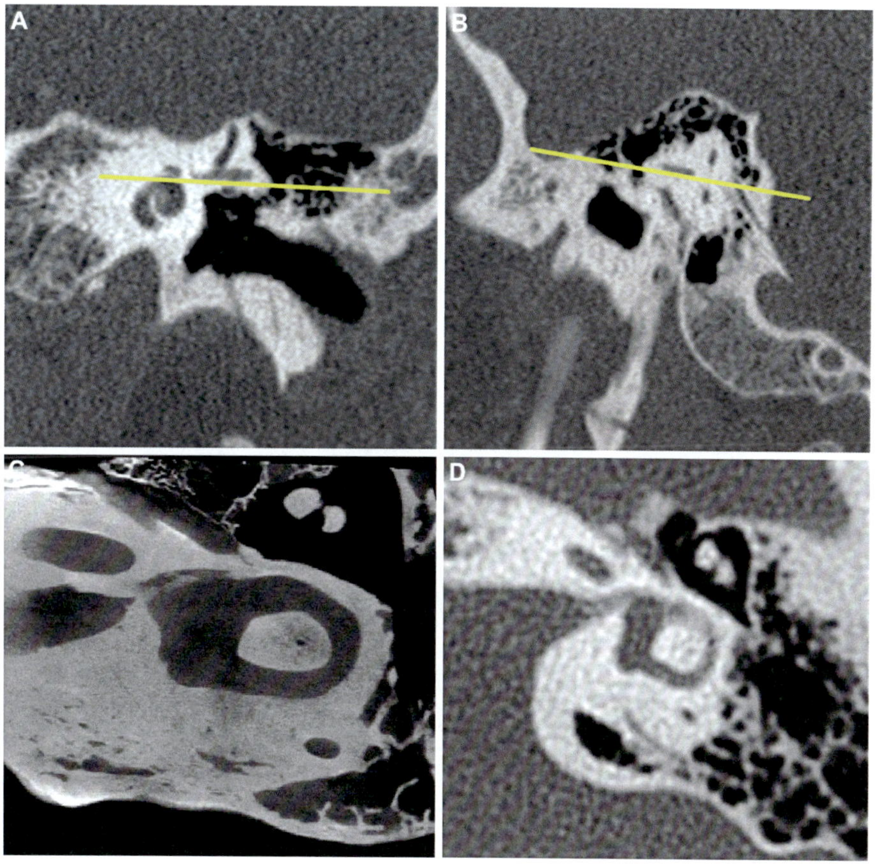

Fig. 31 Oblique axial reconstruction of the lateral semicircular canal. (**a**) Coronal and (**b**) sagittal reference images demonstrating the MPR plane (yellow lines) required for the oblique sagittal view of the lateral semicircular canal. This reconstruction would be unnecessary if standard axial images were reconstructed in the plane of the lateral canal. MPR of the lateral semicircular canal from (**c**) the microCT and (**d**) the MDCT datasets. MPR of the lateral semicircular canal from (**e**) the microMR and (**f**) the 3T MR datasets

Fig. 31 (continued)

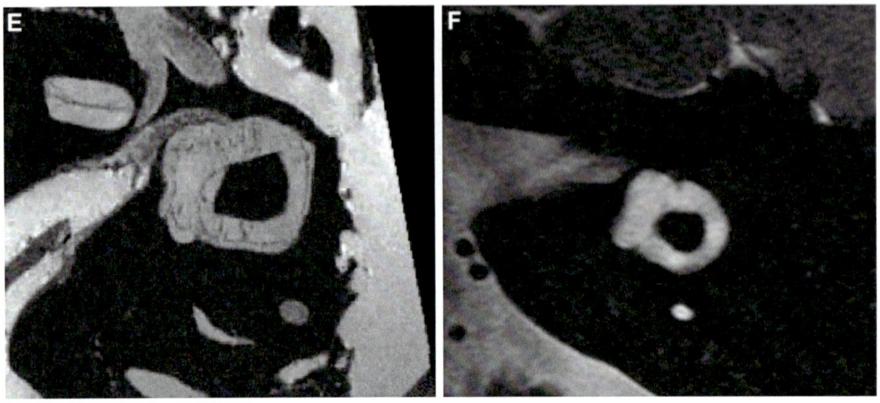

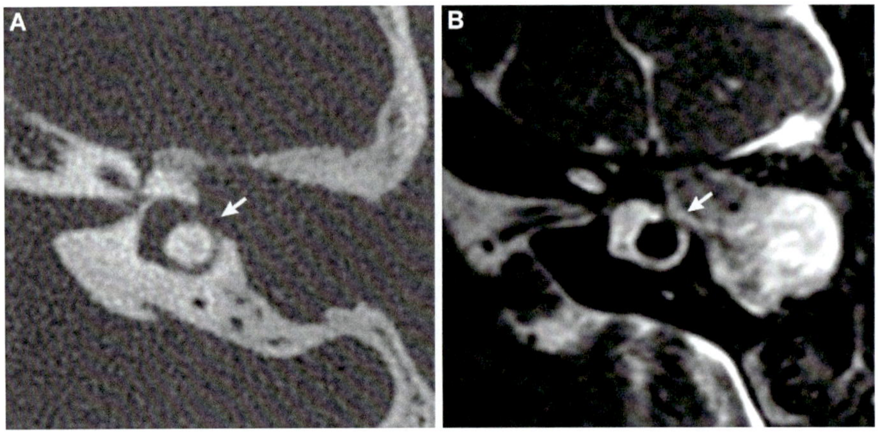

Fig. 32 Clinical application: oblique axial reconstruction of lateral semicircular canal. (**a**) MDCT and (**b**) 3D T2-weighted fast spin-echo 1.5 T reconstruction in patient presenting with positional vertigo related to cholesteatoma with perilymph fistula. Note erosion of the anterior limb of the lateral canal (*arrow*) on both MDCT and 3T MR reconstructions

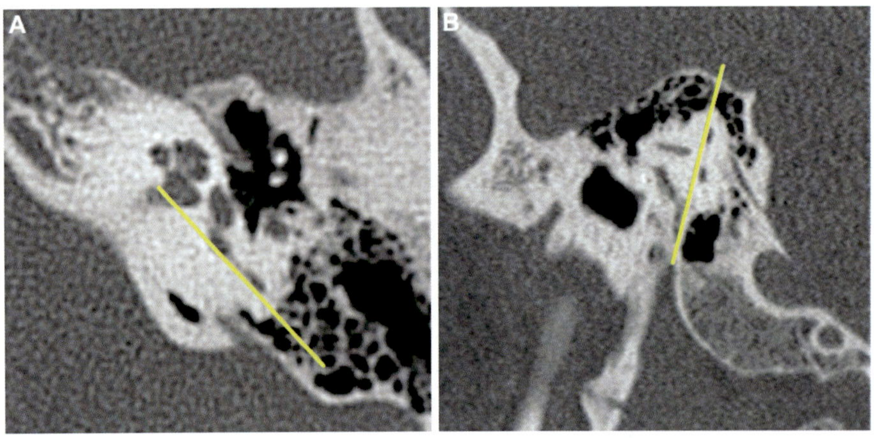

Fig. 33 Oblique coronal reconstruction of the posterior semicircular canal. (**a**) Axial and (**b**) sagittal reference images demonstrating the MPR planes (yellow lines) required for the oblique coronal view of the posterior semicircular canal. This reconstruction is a slight modification of the Stenvers plane. MPR of the posterior semicircular canal from (**c**) the microCT and (**d**) the MDCT datasets. MPR of the posterior semicircular canal from (**e**) the microMR and (**f**) the 3T MR datasets

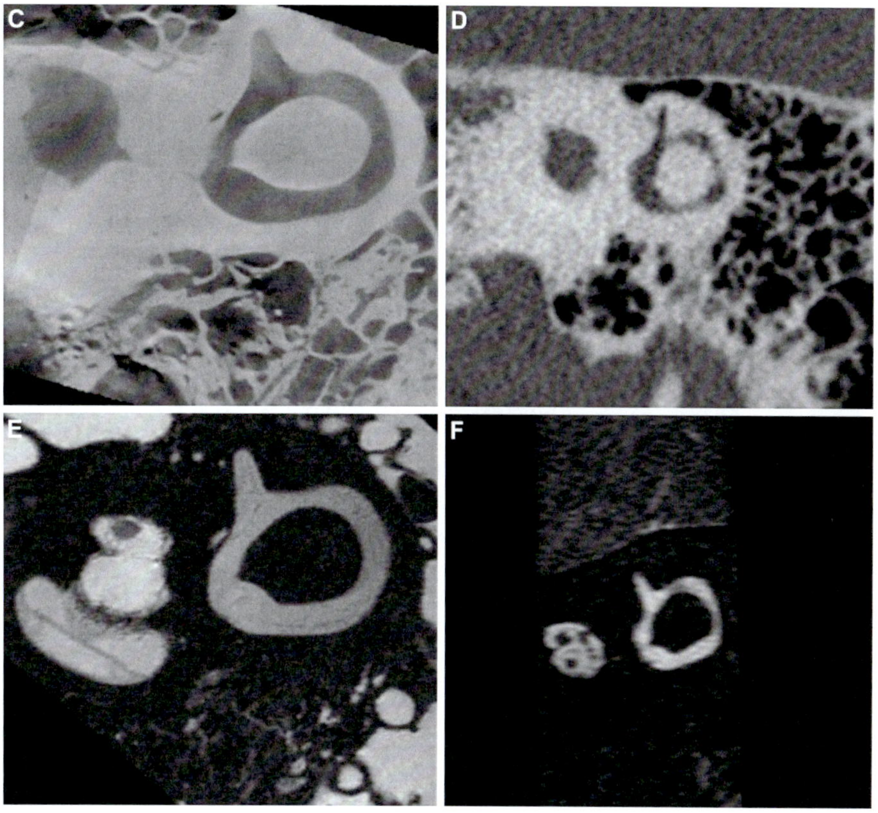

Fig. 33 (continued)

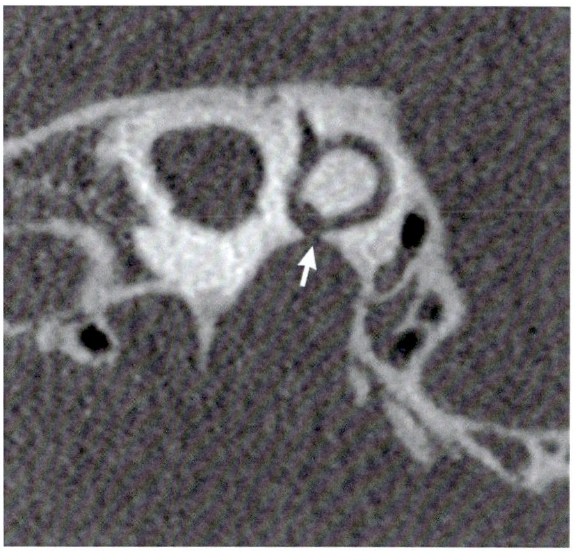

Fig. 34 Clinical application: oblique coronal reconstruction of the posterior semicircular canal. MDCT reconstruction in a patient presenting with vestibular symptoms. Note focal dehiscence of the bony partition between the inferior wall of the ampulla of the posterior semicircular canal (*arrow*) and the adjacent jugular bulb on the MDCT reconstruction

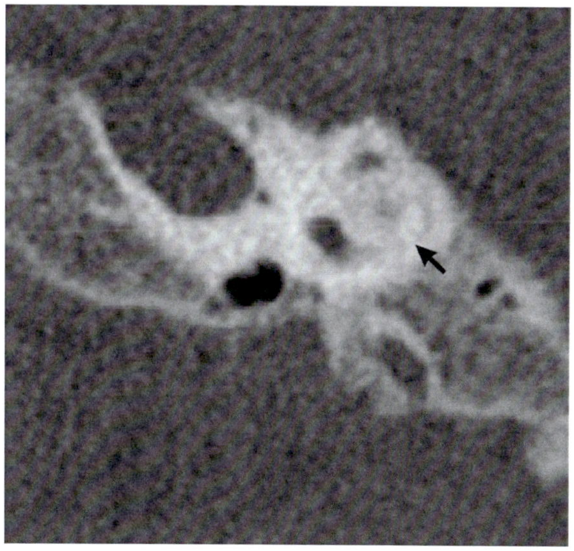

Fig. 35 Clinical application: oblique coronal reconstruction of the posterior semicircular canal. Pre-operative MDCT reconstruction in a patient with profound sensorineural hearing loss as a complication of perinatal meningitis being considered for a cochlear implant. Note labyrinthitis ossificans involving the posterior canal (*arrow*). The basal turn of the cochlea and the lateral canal were also involved

References

1. Hans P, Grant AJ, Laitt RD, Ramsden RT, Kassner A, Jackson A. Comparison of three-dimensional visualization techniques for depicting the scala vestibuli and scala tympani of the cochlea by using high-resolution MR imaging. *AJNR: Am J Neuroradiol* 1999;20:1197–1206
2. Belden CJ, Weg N, Minor LB, Zinreich SJ. CT evaluation of bone dehiscence of the superior semicircular canal as a cause of sound- and/or pressure-induced vertigo. *Radiology* 2003;226: 337–343 [see comment]
3. Henrot P, Iochum S, Batch T, Coffinet L, Blum A, Roland J. Current multiplanar imaging of the stapes. *AJNR: Am J Neuroradiol* 2005;26:2128–2133
4. Lane J, Lindell E, Witte R, DeLone D, Driscoll C. Middle and inner ear: Improved depiction with multiplanar reconstruction of volumetric CT data. *Radiographics* 2006;26:115–124
5. Ozgen B, Cunnane ME, Caruso PA, Curtin HD. Comparison of 45 degrees oblique reformats with axial reformats in CT evaluation of the vestibular aqueduct. *AJNR: Am J Neuroradiol* 2008;29:30–34
6. Bin Z, Jingzhen H, Daocai W, Kai L, Cheng L. Traumatic ossicular chain separation: Sliding-thin-slab maximum-intensity projections for diagnosis. *J Comput Assist Tomogr* 2008;32:951–954
7. Krombach GA, Di Martino E, Martiny S, et al Dehiscence of the superior and/or posterior semicircular canal: Delineation on T2-weighted axial three-dimensional turbo spin-echo images, maximum intensity projections and volume-rendered images. *Eur Arch Otorhinolaryngol* 2006;263: 111–117
8. Naganawa S, Senda K, Yamakawa K, et al [High resolution MR imaging of the inner ear apparatus using 3D-Fast spin echo sequence]. *Nippon Igaku Hoshasen Gakkai Zasshi – Nippon Acta Radiol* 1995;55:81–82

Imaging Microscopy of the Temporal Bone: An Anatomy Tutorial

5

Introduction

The enclosed CD program uses imaging microscopy datasets to construct a computer-based learning module of the middle/inner ear anatomy. T2-weighted microMR images of a cadaver temporal bone specimen scanned on a 9.4 T were acquired at a 78-μm slice thickness after opacification of the middle ear space with dilute gadolinium solution. Images of a second specimen scanned on a microCT unit were acquired at a 20-μm slice thickness. The Temporal Bone Anatomy Tool presents both datasets in orthogonal planes along with a 3D reconstruction (Fig. 1). The Virtual Endoscopy Video Player displays a 3D fly-through sequence composed from the microMR dataset (Fig. 2).

Temporal Bone Anatomy Tool

This tool will display either the microMR or microCT datasets in the axial, sagittal, and coronal planes with the main anatomical structures segmented in colors to match the 3D image displayed in the left upper quadrant.

Datasets may be viewed with the color segmentation on or off by clicking the buttons on the bottom panel. Movement of the reference point in one plane will be automatically co-registered in the other planes. A text box at the bottom of the screen will display the name and definition of each segmented anatomical structure identified by the cursor. This feature may also be turned on or off.

Virtual Endoscopy Video Player

This virtual endoscopic fly-though video can be launched by clicking the "start Movie" button on the face page. The sequence will take the viewer down the left external auditory canal, through the tympanic membrane and into the tympanic space.

The middle ear flight path will continue, passing the tensor tympani tendon and chorda tympani nerve. The camera will then proceed along the posterior wall of the tympanic space identifying the facial recess, pyramidal eminence, stapedius tendon, sinus tympani, and round window niche.

The inner ear sequence will proceed around the cochlea, vestibule, semicircular canals, and the vestibular and cochlear aqueducts. The flight path will continue through the round window membrane into the scala tympani, pass through the spiral lamina into the scala vestibuli, and return back through the basal turn to the vestibule. The camera will then enter the common crus, proceed along the entire posterior semicircular canal, and re-enter the vestibule.

The flight path will exit the inner ear through the oval window, transverse the tympanic space and leave the head by way of the external auditory canal.

J. I. Lane, R. J. Witte, *The Temporal Bone,* DOI: 10.1007/978-3-642-02210-4_5,

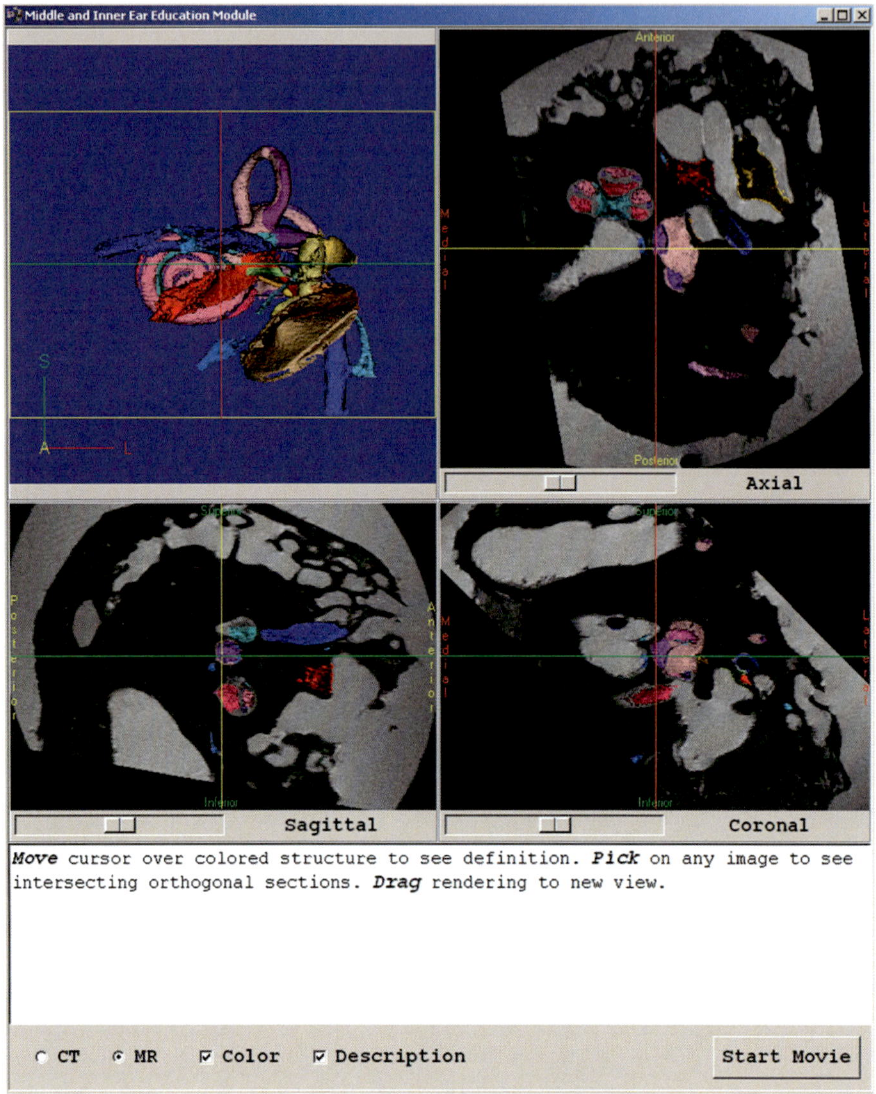

Fig. 1 Screenshot of the user interface for the electronic Temporal Bone Anatomy Tool (see enclosed CD)

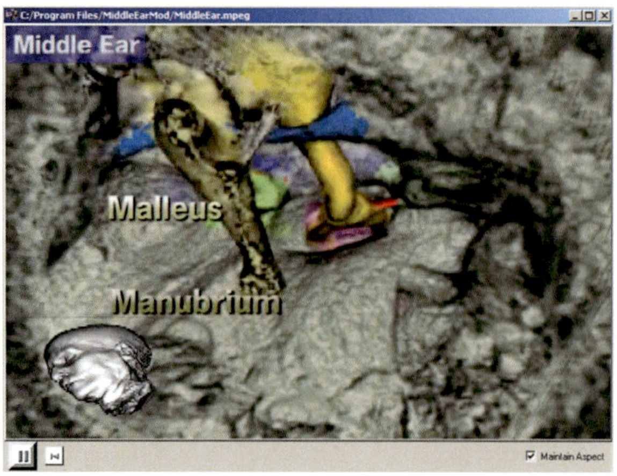

Fig. 2 Screenshot from the Virtual Endoscopy Video Player (see enclosed CD)

Glossary

Aditus ad antrum (AAA) The passage leading from the epitympanic space (attic) to the mastoid antrum.

Ampulla (Am_S, Am_L, Am_P) The expanded ends of the superior, lateral, and posterior semicircular canals that open into the vestibule and contain the neurosensory organs for detection of angular acceleration (see crista ampullaris).

Annular ligament See suspensory ligament, stapedial annular.

Arcuate eminence An anatomical and surgical landmark along the superior surface of the petrous portion of the temporal bone that identifies the location of the superior semicircular canal.

Arnold's nerve Auricular branch of the vagus nerve transmitted from the jugular fossa through the mastoid process by way of the auricular canaliculus; provides the posterior pinna and external auditory canal (EAC) with sensation.

Attic (At) The upper portion of the tympanic cavity above the tympanic membrane; contains the head of the malleus and the body of the incus. Synomyms: epitympanic space, epitympanic recess, epitympanum. See tympanic space.

Auricular canaliculus See Arnold's nerve

Basilar membrane (BM) Stiff layer of mesothelium that separates the endolymphatic cochlear duct from the perilymphatic scala tympani. It extends from the edge of the spiral lamina to the outer wall of the cochlea.

Bill's bar (BB) A vertical bony crest at the lateral end of the IAC, arising from the transverse crest (crista falciformis) that separates the anteriorly situated facial nerve from the more posteriorly situated superior vestibular nerve. Named after renowned neurotologist, Dr. William House.

Carotid canal (CaC) Bony canal that transmits the internal carotid artery through the petrous part of the temporal bone from its inferior surface upward, medially, and forward to the apex.

Chorda tympani (ChT) Branch of the facial (VIIth cranial) nerve that passes through the middle ear between the malleus and incus and continues through the petrotympanic fissure; carries taste sensation from the anterior two-thirds of the tongue and conveys parasympathetic efferents to the salivary glands.

Chorda tympani canal (ChTC) Bony canal transmitting the nerve of the same name; arises from the lateral wall of the distal mastoid segment of the facial nerve canal.

Cochlea (Co_B, Co_M, Co_A) Conch-shaped structure composing the anterior portion of the labyrinth, made up of approximately 2.5 turns or coils (basilar, middle, apical) around the modiolus. Its apex is orientated anteriorly, laterally, and slightly inferiorly.

Cochlear aperture (CoAp) Cribriform opening in the anteroinferior aspect of the internal auditory canal that transmits the branches of the cochlear nerve into the base of the cochlear modiolus.

Cochlear aqueduct (CoAq) A channel containing perilymph passing through the temporal bone, providing potential communication between the scala tympani of the cochlea and the subarachnoid space. It is variably patent in humans.

Cochlear nerve (CoN) The cochlear division of the VIIIth cranial nerve; nerve fibers originate from neurons of the spiral ganglia located within small channels (canals of Rosenthal) at the root of each spiral lamina within the modiolus and project peripherally to cochlear hair cells in the cochlear duct (scala media) and centrally to the cochlear nuclei of the brainstem.

Cochlear promontory (CoP) A bony prominence on the medial wall of the tympanic cavity overlying the lateral margin of the basal turn of the cochlea.

Cochleariform process (CP) A bony angular process above the anterior end of the oval window, forming a pulley over which the tendon of the tensor tympani muscle extends.

Common crus (CC) The united, nonampullary ends of the superior and posterior semicircular ducts and canals.

Crista ampullaris (CrA_S, CrA_L, CrA_P) Neuroepithelial sensory organs that detect angular accleration. They project from the inner surface of the ampulla of each semicircular duct (*s*uperior, *l*ateral, *p*osterior); filaments of the vestibular nerve pass through the crista to reach hair cells on its surface; the hair cells are capped by the cupola, a gelatinous, protein–polysaccharide mass.

Crista falciformis (CF) Horizontal ridge that divides the fundus of the internal auditory canal into a superior and an inferior area. In the former are the opening of the facial canal and openings for the branches of the vestibular nerve to the utricle and to the ampullae of the anterior and lateral semicircular canal. In the latter are openings for the cochlear nerve, and for branches of the vestibular nerve to the saccule and to the ampulla of the posterior semicircular duct. Synonyms: crista transversa, falciform crest, transverse crest.

Ductus reuniens Short, small duct connecting the distal end of the cochlear duct along the floor of the vestibule to the saccule.

Elliptical recess An ellipsoid depression in the anterosuperior aspect of the medial wall of the vestibule that accommodates the utricle.

Endolymph Inner ear fluid with a high potassium content found within the sacs and ducts of the membranous labyrinth; potassium gradient regulates electrochemical impulses of hair cells.

Endolymphatic duct (ED) Duct connecting the endolymphatic sac with the saccule; transmitted by the vestibular aqueduct. It communicates with the endolymph of the utricle by way of the utriculosaccular duct.

Epitympanum See attic and tympanic space.

Eustachian tube (EuT) Tube connecting the pharynx to the middle ear space allowing for equalization of pressure across the eardrum; opens along the anterior wall of the tympanic space inferior to the semi canal of the tensor tympani. Synonym: auditory tube.

Facial nerve (FN_L, FN_T, FN_M) Nerve that originates in the dorsal pons, passes through the internal auditory canal, and courses through the temporal bone in three segments (labyrinthine, tympanic, mastoid); contains three types of nerve fibers: (1) motor fibers to the superficial muscles of the face, neck, and scalp and the muscles of facial expression; (2) sensory fibers, carrying impulses from the taste sensors in the anterior two-thirds of the tongue and general sensory impulses from tissues adjacent to the tongue; and (3) parasympathetic fibers (autonomic) to the ganglia governing the lacrimal glands and certain salivary glands.

Facial nerve canal (FNC_L, FNC_T, FNC_M) Bony canal transmitting the facial nerve through the temporal bone: composed of three segments (labyrinthine, tympanic, mastoid); the labyrinthine segment commences at the lateral end of the internal auditory canal and passes anteriorly to the geniculate ganglion (first genu), the tympanic segment then turns posteriorly to pass beneath the lateral semicircular canal along the medial wall of the tympanic cavity, and finally, the mastoid segment turns inferiorly (second genu) and descends to reach the stylomastoid foramen. Synonym: ??fallopian canal.

Facial recess (FR) Recess along the posterior wall of the tympanic space that is lateral to the mastoid segment of the facial nerve canal and pyramidal eminence and medial to the chorda tympani nerve; site of surgical entry into the tympanic space from the mastoid approach.

Fissula ante fenestram Minute, slit-like cleft in the otic labyrinthine wall anterior to the oval window of the vestibule. The bone around it often contains fibrous tissue and immature cartilage. This site has a predilection for otosclerosis and for some perilymphatic fistulae.

Fossa incudis (FoI) A small depression in the lower and posterior part of the attic (epitympanic space) that contains the short limb of the incus.

Geniculate ganglion (GG) The L-shaped collection of fibers and sensory neurons of the facial nerve located at the junction of the labyrinthine and tympanic segments of the facial nerve canal. It receives fibers from the motor, sensory, and parasympathetic components of the facial nerve and sends fibers that will innervate the lacrimal glands, submandibular glands, sublingual glands, tongue, palate, pharynx, EAC, stapedius, posterior belly of the digastric muscle, stylohyoid muscle, and muscles of facial expression. Sensory and parasympathetic inputs are carried into the geniculate ganglion via the nervus intermedius. Motor fibers are carried via the facial nerve proper. The greater superficial petrosal nerve, which carries sensory fibers as well as preganglionic parasympathetic fibers, emerges from the anterior aspect of the ganglion.

Helicotrema See scala vestibuli.

Hypotympanum See tympanic space.

Incus (In_B, In_L, In_{Le}, In_S) One of three ossicles in the ear lying between the malleus and stapes. The incus consists of a body and two processes. The body (In_B) is somewhat cubical, but compressed transversely. On its anterior surface is a deeply concavo-convex facet that articulates with the head of the malleus. The two processes diverge at right angles from one another. The short crus or process (In_S), somewhat conical in shape, projects almost horizontally backward, and is attached to the fossa incudis, in the lower and posterior parts of the attic (epitympanic space). The long process (In_L) descends nearly vertically behind and parallel to the manubrium of the malleus, and, bending medialward, ends in a rounded projection, the lenticular process (In_{Le}), which is tipped with cartilage, and articulates with the head of the stapes.

Inferior vestibular nerve (IVN_S, IVN_P) Division of the vestibular nerve composed of two branches that innervate the saccule and ampulla of the posterior semicircular canal. The saccular branch (IVN_S) exits the IAC through a small canal and ends in the saccular macula; the posterior branch (IVN_P) runs through the singular canal and supplies the ampulla of the posterior semicircular duct.

Inferior vestibular nerve canal (IVNC) A short bony canal or foramen transmitting the saccular branch of the inferior vestibular nerve from the IAC to a small area of cribriform bone (area vestibularis inferior) in the spherical recess of the medial wall of the vestibule.

Internal auditory canal (IAC) Bony canal in the petrous bone, between the structures of the inner ear and the cerebellopontine angle. It contains the vestibulocochlear nerve (branching in the canal into the cochlear nerve, and the superior and inferior vestibular nerves) and the facial nerve.

Interscalar septum(a) (IS) Bony partitions separating the turns of the cochlea. They connect the modiolus to the otic capsule.

Jacobson's nerve A nerve from the inferior ganglion of the glossopharygeal nerve; it enters the temporal bone just anterior to the jugular foramen and is transmitted by the tympanic canaliculus to the middle ear where it forms the tympanic plexus on the surface of the cochlear promontory, supplying sensation to the mucus membrane of the tympanic cavity, mastoid cells, and Eustachian tube; presynaptic parasympathetic fibers also pass through the tympanic nerve via the lesser superficial petrosal nerve to the otic ganglion, where they synapse with postsynaptic fibers that continue to supply the parotid gland.

Jugular foramen/fossa (JF) A passage between the petrous portion of the temporal bone and the jugular process of the occipital bone, sometimes divided into two by the jugular spine; it contains the internal jugular vein, inferior petrosal sinus, the glossopharyngeal, vagus, and spinal accessory nerves, and the meningeal branches of the ascending pharyngeal and occipital arteries.

Labyrinth The inner ear; it is composed of an inner membranous portion and outer bony portion.

Lenticular process (In_{Le}) See incus

Ligament See Suspensory Ligaments

Malleus (Ma_A, Ma_H, Ma_L, Ma_M, Ma_N) One of three ossicles in the ear; consists of a head, neck, and three processes: the manubrium, the anterior process and the lateral process. The head (Ma_H) is the large upper extremity of the bone; it is oval in shape, and articulates posteriorly with the incus. The facet for articulation with the incus is constricted near the middle, and consists of an upper larger and lower smaller part. The neck (Ma_N) is the narrow, contracted part just beneath the head. The manubrium (Ma_M) is connected with the tympanic membrane by its lateral margin. It is directed downward, medialward, and backward; it decreases in size toward its free end, which is curved slightly forward, and flattened transversely. The tendon of the tensor tympani inserts on its medial surface, near its upper end. The anterior process (Ma_A) is a delicate spicule below the neck projecting anteriorly and connected to the petrotympanic fissure by delicate membranes. The lateral process (Ma_L) is a conical projection, emanating from the root of the manubrium; it is directed laterally, and is attached to the upper part of the tympanic membrane and to the edges of the notch of Rivinus by the anterior and posterior malleolar folds.

Manubrium (Ma_M) See malleus.

Mastoid antrum (MA) Cavity in the petrous portion of the temporal bone, communicating posteriorly with the mastoid air cells and anteriorly with the attic (epitympanic space) of the middle ear via the aditus ad antrum.

Mesotympanum See tympanic space.

Modiolus (Mo) The central column in the osseous cochlea composed of cribriform bone accommodating the fibers of the cochlear nerve.

Notch of Rivinus Deficiency/notch in the (tympanic annular) ring of connective tissue that holds the tympanic membrane in place. This defect produces the focal laxity known as the pars flaccida of the tympanic membrane. Named after Augustus Quirinus Rivinus, eighteenth century German physician and professor of pathology.

Otic capsule Dense bone encasing the inner ear structures within the petrous portion of the temporal bone.

Oval window (OW) An oval opening in the medial wall of the middle ear leading into the vestibule covered by the footplate of the stapes.

Pars flaccida See tympanic membrane.

Pars tensa See tympanic membrane.

Perilymph Inner ear fluid that surrounds the membranous sacs and ducts of the labyrinth; chemical composition is similar to that of cerebrospinal fluid.

Pinna The external ear; skin-covered cartilaginous funnel-shaped appendage centered at the EAC.

Ponticulus See sinus tympani.

Porus acusticus Opening of the internal auditory canal on the posterior surface of the petrous portion of the temporal bone.

Prussak's space (PS) Small middle ear recess, bordered laterally by the pars flaccida of the tympanic membrane, superiorly by the scutum and lateral mallear ligament, inferiorly by the lateral process of the malleus, and medially by the neck of the malleus; commonly occupied by pars flaccida cholesteatomata. It is named after the Russian otologist, Alexander Prussak (1839–1897).

Pyramidal eminence (PE) A conical projection from the posterior wall of the middle ear posterior to the oval window; it is hollow and contains the stapedius muscle and tendon.

Reissner's membrane (RM) Membrane that separates the scala media from the scala vestibuli. Together with the basilar membrane it defines the space occupied by the cochlear duct within the scala media, which contains the organ of Corti. It primarily functions as a diffusion barrier, allowing nutrients to travel from the perilymph to the endolymph of the membranous labyrinth. Named after the German anatomist, Ernst Reissner (1824–1878).

Rosenthal's canal See cochlear nerve

Round window (RW) Membrane at the basal end of the scala tympani that bulges out to accommodate perilymph fluid displacement at the oval window. It allows fluid in the cochlea to move, stimulating the hair cells of the basilar membrane. The round window is situated inferior and posterior to the oval window, separated by the cochlear promontory.

Round window niche (RWN) A funnel-shaped depression in the medial wall of the middle ear into which the round window opens.

Saccular macula (SaM) The neuroepithelial sensory receptor along the anteromedial wall of the saccule composed of a statoconial membrane supported by hair cells to which the saccular filaments of the inferior vestibular nerve are distributed; the vertical plane of orientation is perpendicular to that of the utricular macula.

Saccule (Sa) Smaller of the two endolymphatic vestibular sacs; it is spherical in form, and lies in the spherical recess near the opening of the scala vestibuli of the cochlea. It functions in concert with the utricle to detect linear acceleration.

Scala media (SM) Spiral endolymphatic tube lying within the outer wall of the bony cochlea; it is separated from the perilymphatic scala vestibuli by Reissner's membrane and from the perilymphatic scala tympani by the basilar membrane. Synonym: cochlear duct.

Scala tympani (ST) Spiral perilymphatic tube lying within the lumen of the cochlea located posterior to the spiral lamina; its basilar end terminates at the round window.

Scala vestibuli (SV) Spiral perilymphatic tube lying within the lumen of the cochlea located anterior to the spiral lamina; its basilar end opens into the floor of the vestibule by way of an oval-shaped aperture; transmits a perilymphatic fluid wave generated at the oval window into the cochlea; communicates with the scala tympani by way of a small defect at the apex of the cochlea, the helicotrema.

Scarpa's ganglion See vestibular nerve.

Scutum (Sc) A sharp bony spur formed by the lateral wall of the tympanic cavity and the superior wall of the EAC. Its inferior edge is part of the bony ridge to which the tympanic membrane is attached. The scutum becomes eroded at an early stage by pars flaccida cholesteatoma.

Semi canal of the tensor tympani (SeC) Incomplete bony canal containing the tensor tympani muscle and separating it from the Eustachian tube inferiorly along the anterior wall of the tympanic space.

Semicircular canal (SCC_S, SCC_L, SCC_P) Tubular canals within the bony labyrinth that contain perilymph and transmit the endolymphatic semicircular ducts, which are attached to the outer walls of the canals. The three canals (superior, lateral, posterior) are set at right angles to each other and communicate with the vestibule through five openings, one of which is common to the nonampullated limbs of the superior and posterior canals (common crus). Each canal has an ampullated end in which the cristae ampullaris of the corresponding duct is situated.

Semicircularduct(SCD_S, SCD_L, SCD_P) Endolymph-filled tubes attached to the outer walls of the semicircular canals, each of which has an ampullated end containing the crista ampullaris, the neurosensory organ responsible for detecting angular or rotational acceleration. The ducts occupy about one-fourth of the volume of the canals, the remainder being filled with perilymph. Each duct communicates with the utricle. The superior and posterior ducts share a common limb (common crus) resulting in five orifices opening into the utricle from the three ducts (superior, lateral, posterior).

Singular canal (SiC) Bony canal that transmits the posterior branch of the inferior vestibular nerve from the ampulla of the posterior semicircular canal to the posteroinferior border of the internal auditory canal.

Sinus tympani (SiT) Small recess located between the medial wall of the tympanic space and the pyramidal eminence; common site for the extension or recurrence of pars tensa cholesteatoma; often obscured by the pyramidal eminence at surgery (tympanomastoidectomy approach). It is separated from the oval window by an anterior bony ridge, the ponticulus, and from the round window niche by an inferior bony ridge, the subiculum.

Spherical recess A rounded depression along the anteroinferior aspect of the medial wall of the vestibule that accommodates the saccule.

Spiral lamina (SL) An incomplete bony shelf projecting from the modiolus; along with the basilar membrane it separates the scala tympani from the scala vestibuli and scala media.

Stapedial muscle (StM) Muscle that is transmitted through the hollow center of the pyramidal eminence innervated by a branch of the facial nerve. Its reflex contractions tend to tip the stapes backward, as if to pull it out of the oval window. It selectively reduces the intensity of sounds entering the inner ear, especially those of lower frequency.

Stapedial tendon (StT) Tendon of the stapedial muscle that extends from the hollow center of the pyramidal eminence to its attachment on the posterior surface of the neck of the stapes; responsible for the reflex dampening of stapes vibrations during exposure to loud sound. See stapedial muscle.

Stapes (St_H, St_N, St_P, St_A, St_F) One of three ossicles in the ear; consists of a head, neck, anterior crus, posterior crus, and footplate. The head (St_H) articulates with the lenticular process of the incus. The short neck (St_N) receives the stapedial tendon onto its posterior surface. Of the two crura, the posterior crus (St_P) is thicker and has less of a curvature than the more grassile, bowed anterior crus (St_A). The kidney-shaped footplate (St_F) is convex superiorly, concave inferiorly, and fixed to the inner edge of the oval window by the annular ligament.

Stylomastoid foramen of the facial nerve Point of exit of the mastoid segment of the facial nerve found between the styloid and mastoid processes on the inferior surface of the temporal bone.

Subiculum See sinus tympani.

Superior vestibular nerve (SVN) Division of the vestibular nerve that innervates the utricular macula and ampullae of the superior and lateral semicircular ducts; exits the IAC through a short bony canal and its fibers pass through a small area of cribriform bone (area vestibularis superior) that includes the vestibular pyramid in the anterior wall of the vestibule.

Superior vestibular nerve canal (SVNC) Short bony canal that transmits the superior division of the vestibular nerve from the IAC to the anterior wall of the vestibule where nerve fibers pass through a small area of cribriform bone (area vestibularis superior) to innervate the utricular macula and ampullae of the superior and lateral semicircular ducts.

Suspensory ligaments Delicate, fibrous bands that stabilize the auditory ossicles with in the middle ear cavity. The six ligaments consist of the:

- **Mallear anterior (LMA)** Anterior mallear ligament; suspensory ligament attached by one end to the neck of the malleus, just above the anterior process, and by the other to the anterior wall of the tympanic cavity, close to the petrotympanic fissure.
- **Mallear lateral (LML)** Lateral mallear ligament; suspensory ligament composed of a triangular fibrous band passing from the posterior part of the notch of Rivinus to the head of the malleus.
- **Mallear superior (LMS)** Superior mallear ligament; delicate suspensory ligament that descends from the roof of the epitympanic space to the head of the malleus.
- **Incudal posterior (LIP)** Posterior incudal ligament; short, thick suspensory ligament connecting the end of the short process of the incus to the fossa incudis.
- **Incudal superior (LIS)** Superior incudal ligament; little more than a fold of mucous membrane that descends from the roof of the epitympanic recess to the body of the incus.
- **Stapedial annular (LSA)** Annular stapedial ligament; a fibrous ring that attaches the stapes footplate to the margins of the oval window.

Tegmen tympani (TeT) Thin bony roof of the attic (epitympanic space) and mastoid antrum.

Tensor tympani (TT) Muscle that emerges from a bony semi canal just above the opening of the Eustachian tube and runs posteriorly over a pulley-like projection of bone, the cochleariform process, and then laterally to attach to the upper part of the manubrium of the malleus. It acts in a reflex manner to dampen sound conduction, protecting the inner ear from acoustic injury. When contracted, the tensor tympani pulls the malleus inward and increases the tension of the tympanic membrane, particularly with chewing. It is innervated by a branch of the mandibular division of the Vth cranial nerve arising from the otic ganglion.

Tympanic canaliculus See Jacobson's nerve.

Tympanic membrane (TM) A thin, semitransparent membrane separating the EAC from the tympanic space; its outer circumference forms a fibrocartilaginous ring that is fixed at the inner edge of the EAC in the tympanic sulcus. This sulcus is deficient superiorly (notch of Rivinus). The triangular segment of the TM adjacent to the notch is lax and thin (pars flaccida); the remainder is thick and taut (pars tensa). Its manubrial attachment draws the TM medially toward the tympanic space, producing a concave lateral surface of the TM, the most depressed part of which is called the umbo.

Tympanic space Middle ear space; it can be divided into the epitympanum, mesotympanum, and hypotympanum. The epitympanum or attic is the portion of the middle ear that is above the roof of the EAC and contains the head of the malleus and body/short process of the incus. The mesotympanum is the portion between the roof and floor of the EAC, much of which is visible through the normal tympanic membrane. The hypotympanum is the portion of the middle ear below the floor of the EAC that contains the opening of the Eustachian tube anteriorly.

Umbo See tympanic membrane.

Utricular macula (UtM) The neuroepithelial sensory receptor in the anteroinferior wall of the utricle composed of a statoconial membrane supported by hair cells to which the utricular filaments of the superior vestibular nerve are distributed. It lies in a horizontal plane perpendicular to the saccular macula and acts in concert with the saccule to detect linear acceleration.

Utricle (Ut) Larger of the two endolymphatic vestibular sacs; it is ellipsoid in form, and lies in the elliptical recess above the vestibular crest, which separates it from the saccule below. It functions in concert with the saccule to detect linear acceleration.

Utriculosaccular duct Small duct that connects the utricle with the endolymphatic duct a short distance from its connection with the saccule.

Vestibular aqueduct (VA) Bony canal transmitting the endolymphatic duct; it has its origin in a small orifice in the posteromedial wall of the vestibule, just anterior to the orifice of the common crus, and extends posteroinferiorly to the posterior surface of the petrous portion of the temporal bone.

Vestibular crest (VC) Bony ridge separating the elliptical (utricular) recess from the spherical (saccular) recess along the medial wall of the vestibule.

Vestibular nerve One of two major trunks of the VIIIth cranial nerve made up of two divisions, the inferior and superior vestibular nerves (see inferior vestibular nerve and superior vestibular nerve); composed of bipolar cells originating from Scarpa's ganglion found within the fundus of the internal auditory canal.

Vestibular pyramid (VP) Superior termination of the vestibular crest composed of elevated cribriform bone transmitting the utricular fibers of the superior vestibular nerve to the utricular macula.

Vestibule (V) The central part of the osseous labyrinth, situated medial to the tympanic cavity, posterior to the cochlea; it receives the limbs of the semicircular canals, opens anteroinferiorly into the scala vestibuli of the cochlea, and contains the saccule and utricle.

Vestibulocochlear nerve Eighth cranial nerve carrying acoustic and vestibular impulses from the inner ear.

Index

A
Analyze 3D voxel registration program, 1
Annular ligament, 11, 99
Arcuate eminence, 8
Arnold's nerve, 99
Attic, 10, 99
Auditory ossicle, 11
Axial plane, 30, 31

B
Basilar membrane, 21, 99
Bill's bar, 23, 27, 99
Bone surface, 7–8
Bony external auditory canal, 9
Bony labyrinth, 2, 5

C
Carotid canal, 99
Charge-couple device (CCD) camera, 1
Cholesteatoma, 94
Chorda tympani, 99
  nerve, 11, 97
Cochlea, 12, 17, 83–87, 99
  modiolus, 89, 90
Cochlear
  aperture, 99
  aqueduct, 7, 19, 24, 99
  duct, 12
  implant, 95
  nerve, 23, 100
    hiatus, 84, 85
  promontory, 100
Cochleariform process, 100
Common crus, 18, 100
Computed tomography (CT), 75
  microscopy (*see* Micro CT)
Computer-based learning, 97
Congenital ossicular anomaly, 76
Constructive interference in steady state (CISS), 3
Coronal plane, 40, 41
Crista
  ampullaris, 17, 100
  falciformis, 23, 100

D
Disarticulated ossicles, 13–15
Ductus reuniens, 100

E
EAC. *See* External auditory canal
Elliptical recess, 17, 100
Endolymph, 2, 11, 100
Endolymphatic
  duct, 18, 100
  sac, 19
Epitympanum, 9, 11
Eustachian tube, 11, 100
External auditory canal (EAC), 7, 97
External ear, 7

F
Facial nerve, 87, 100
  canal, 25, 51, 64, 100
  stylomastoid foramen, 104
Facial recess, 100
Fast spin-echo (FSE), 3
Fenesteral otospongiosis, 82, 83
Fissula antefenestrum, 82, 83, 100
Fossa incudis, 101

G
Geniculate ganglion, 101

H
Helicotrema, 20
High field magnetic resonance, 2
Hypoplastic middle ear, 78
Hypotympanum, 9

I
IAC. *See* Internal auditory canal
Imaging microscopy, 1
Incus, 11, 76–79, 81, 101
Inferior vestibular nerve, 23, 101
  canal, 102
Inner ear, 11, 16–19, 76
  disease, 79
Internal auditory canal (IAC), 4, 7, 23–25, 27, 101
Interscalar septum, 84, 101

Isotropic
  volumetric acquisitions, 29
  voxel size, 75

J

Jacobson's nerve, 9, 101
Jugular foramen/fossa, 11, 101

L

Labyrinth, 11, 101
  anomalies, 79
  lateral wall, 22
  medial wall, 22
Labyrinthitis ossificans, 79, 84, 89, 95
Lateral semicircular canal, 30, 40, 93–95
Long axis plane of temporal bone, 64

M

Magnetic resonance
  high field, 2
  microscopy, 1, 2 (*see also* MicroMR)
Malleus, 9, 11, 75–79, 81, 102
  manubrium, 80
Manubrium, 9, 80
Mastoid antrum, 10, 102
Maximum intensity projection (MIP), 3, 76
MDCT. *See* Multidetector CT
Membranous labyrinth, 3, 4, 17
  endolymphatic compartment, 12
Mesotympanum, 9
MicroCT, 1, 4
MicroMR, 4
Microtia, 78
Middle ear, 10, 76
  lateral wall, 11
  posteromedial wall, 10
Modiolus, 102
  of the cochlea, 89, 90
Mondini malformation, 85, 90
Multidetector CT (MDCT), 2, 29, 75
Multiplanar reconstruction (MPR), 3, 76

N

Navicular fossa, 7
Notch of Rivinus, 9, 10, 102

O

Ossicle, 76
Otic capsule, 12, 102
  ossicles, 12
Otospongiotic lesion, 79
Oval window, 20, 102

P

Pars
  flaccida, 9, 10
  tensa, 9
    cholesteatoma, 10
Perilymph/perilymphatic, 2, 11, 21, 102
  compartment, 19
  fistula, 94
  space, 16, 18
Perinatal meningitis, 95
Pinna, 7, 102
Polytomography, 2, 29, 75
Porus acusticus, 24, 102
Pöschl plane, 3, 29, 51, 52, 76, 79
Postprocessing, 3
Prussak's space, 10, 102
Pyramidal eminence, 10, 102

R

Reissner's membrane, 21, 102
Rosenthal's canal, 23
Round window, 102

S

Saccular macula, 103
Saccule, 12, 103
Scala
  media, 103
  tympani, 20, 21, 83, 84, 89, 97, 103
  vestibuli, 20, 83, 97, 103
Scarpa's ganglion, 23
Scutum, 10, 103
Semicircular duct, 17, 103
Sensorineural hearing loss, 90, 91, 95
Short axis plane of temporal bone, 51
Singular canal, 24, 103
Sinus tympani, 10, 103
Skin surface, 7
Specific absorption rate (SAR), 3
Spherical recess, 17, 104
Spiral lamina, 20, 104
Stapedial
  muscle, 104
  tendon, 104
Stapes, 11, 81–83, 104
Stenvers plane, 3, 29, 64, 65, 86, 94
Stylomastoid foramen of the facial nerve, 104
Superior
  semicircular canal, 92, 93
  vestibular nerve, 23, 25, 104
Suspensory ligaments, 11, 104

T

Tegmen tympani, 8, 9, 104
Temporal bone
  anatomy, 7
  anatomy tool, 97, 98
  imaging, 1
    historical perspectives, 29
  inferior surface, 8
  lateral surface, 8
  posteromedial surface, 8
  superior surface, 8
  trauma, 76
Tensor tympani, 11, 104
  semicanal, 11, 103
  tendon, 97
Tullio's phenomenon, 93

Tympanic
canaliculus, 9
membrane, 9, 105
space, 9, 105
Tympanosclerosis, 76
Tympanostomy tube, 78

U
Umbo, 9
Utricle, 12, 105
Utricular macula, 12, 105
Utriculosaccular duct, 18, 105

V
Variable flip angle fast spin-echo (VFA FSE), 3
Vertigo, 93
Vestibular
aqueduct, 7, 18, 19, 24, 90, 91, 105
crest, 17, 23, 105
nerve, 23, 105
pyramid, 105
Vestibule, 105
Vestibulocochlear nerve, 23, 105
Virtual endoscopy video player, 97, 98

W
Wobbling focal spot, 2

X
X-ray, 1

FSC
www.fsc.org
MIX
Papier | Fördert gute Waldnutzung
FSC® C083411

Kolibri 360 GmbH
Ferdinand-Jühlke-Straße 7
99095 Erfurt, Deutschland
produktsicherheit@kolibri360.de